AF877868

Post COVID-19 - Effects on Human Health

Edited by Nicolás Padilla-Raygoza

Published in London, United Kingdom

Post COVID-19 - Effects on Human Health
http://dx.doi.org/10.5772/intechopen.105656
Edited by Nicolás Padilla-Raygoza

Scientific contributor: Mayank Vats

Contributors
Thajus Asirvatham, Premraj Isaac Chandran, Ajay Boppana, Teodora Safiye, Ardea Milidrag, Said Čekić, Draško Dubljanin, Andreja Kovačević, Milena Zlatanović, Merdin Markišić, Mile Despotović, Medo Gutić, Mohammed Somaili, Maja Kuzmanovic, Klaus Meier, Agnieszka Bienert, Felipe Yagnam Rojas, Martina Smolic, Reham Dawood, Ghada Salum, Mai Abd El Meguid, Moataza Omran, Robert Smolic, Nicolás Padilla-Raygoza, Efrain Navarro-Olivos, Gilberto Flores-Vargas, Guadalupe Irazú Morales-Reyes, Jessica Paola Plascencia-Roldán, Maria de Jesús Gallardo-Luna

© The Editor(s) and the Author(s) 2023

The rights of the editor(s) and the author(s) have been asserted in accordance with the Copyright, Designs and Patents Act 1988. All rights to the book as a whole are reserved by INTECHOPEN LIMITED. The book as a whole (compilation) cannot be reproduced, distributed or used for commercial or non-commercial purposes without INTECHOPEN LIMITED's written permission. Enquiries concerning the use of the book should be directed to INTECHOPEN LIMITED rights and permissions department (permissions@intechopen.com).

Violations are liable to prosecution under the governing Copyright Law.

(cc) BY

Individual chapters of this publication are distributed under the terms of the Creative Commons Attribution 3.0 Unported License which permits commercial use, distribution and reproduction of the individual chapters, provided the original author(s) and source publication are appropriately acknowledged. If so indicated, certain images may not be included under the Creative Commons license. In such cases users will need to obtain permission from the license holder to reproduce the material. More details and guidelines concerning content reuse and adaptation can be found at http://www.intechopen.com/copyright-policy.html.

Notice

Statements and opinions expressed in the chapters are these of the individual contributors and not necessarily those of the editors or publisher. No responsibility is accepted for the accuracy of information contained in the published chapters. The publisher assumes no responsibility for any damage or injury to persons or property arising out of the use of any materials, instructions, methods or ideas contained in the book.

First published in London, United Kingdom, 2023 by IntechOpen
IntechOpen is the global imprint of INTECHOPEN LIMITED, registered in England and Wales, registration number: 11086078, 5 Princes Gate Court, London, SW7 2QJ, United Kingdom

British Library Cataloguing-in-Publication Data
A catalogue record for this book is available from the British Library

Additional hard and PDF copies can be obtained from orders@intechopen.com

Post COVID-19 - Effects on Human Health
Edited by Nicolás Padilla-Raygoza
p. cm.
Print ISBN 978-1-83768-487-8
Online ISBN 978-1-83768-488-5
eBook (PDF) ISBN 978-1-83768-489-2

We are IntechOpen, the world's leading publisher of Open Access books

Built by scientists, for scientists

6,400+
Open access books available

174,000+
International authors and editors

190M+
Downloads

156
Countries delivered to

Our authors are among the
Top 1%
most cited scientists

12.2%
Contributors from top 500 universities

CLARIVATE ANALYTICS BOOK CITATION INDEX INDEXED

WEB OF SCIENCE™

Selection of our books indexed in the Book Citation Index in Web of Science™ Core Collection (BKCI)

Interested in publishing with us?
Contact book.department@intechopen.com

Numbers displayed above are based on latest data collected.
For more information visit www.intechopen.com

Meet the editor

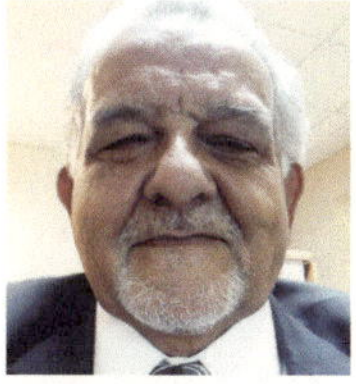

Dr. Nicolás Padilla-Raygoza was Professor Titular B, Department of Nursing and Obstetrics, Division of Health Sciences and Engineering, Campus Celaya-Salvatierra, University of Guanajuato, Mexico, and Coordinator of Research and Continuous Education, School of Medicine, University of Celaya, México. He is currently a coordinator of research projects at the Institute of Public Health, Guanajuato State. He obtained an MD from the Autonomous University of Guadalajara School of Medicine, National Autonomous University of Mexico (UAG-UNAM) in 1984, a specialization in pediatrics from the Mexican Council of Certification in 1986, a postgraduate degree in Epidemiology from the University of London in 2001, a master's degree and doctorate degree in Science from Atlantic International University (AIU) in 2006, and a master's degree in Social Gerontology from the International Iberoamerican University (UNINI Mexico) in 2017. Dr. Padilla-Raygoza has 169 journal articles and 48 book chapters to his credit. He has also edited four books on health. He was recognized as a state researcher on health by the Institute of Public Health, Guanajuato State in 2015 and as a researcher with social impact by the National Council on Science and Technology (CoNaCyT) in 2016. He was previously a member of the National Researchers System and is a current member of CoNaCyT, Mexico, and the Mexican Academy of Pediatrics. He is also a fellow of the Royal Society of Public Health.

Contents

Preface

The COVID-19 pandemic has had myriad negative consequences around the globe. As of December 2022, there were 649,038,437 confirmed cases and 6,645,812 deaths worldwide. In Mexico, for example, there were 7,222,611 confirmed cases and 331,030 deaths [1].

The pandemic caused much fear, especially when secondary effects such as anosmia, dysgeusia, coagulation disorders, stroke, and cardiovascular problems that could lead to death began to be reported. In addition, there were reports of other sequelae such as pulmonary fibrosis, mental disorders, kidney problems, and more. This book provides a comprehensive overview of post-COVID effects on human health. Chapter 1 discusses treatments of COVID-19 and vaccines and examines their relationship to post-COVID sequelae. Chapter 2 examines Multisystemic Inflammatory Syndrome in children (MIS-c); it was very important in children with COVID-19. Post-COVID-19 stroke and rehabilitation were reviewed in Chapter 3.

The relationship between mental health and COVID-19 was reviewed and analysed in Chapter 4; it is suggested that mental health in the aftermath of the pandemic should be closely monitored. This issue was very important because the threat of being infected by SARS-CoV-2 generated a lot of fear in the world population. In addition to those who were infected, anguish and emotional disorders were generated due to the fear of facing a serious illness or death and in those around them, isolation and not performing the usual tasks also cause disturbances in mental health. Chapter 5 reviewed hydro electrolytic alterations that could be mediated by antidiuretic hormones. Chapter 6 presents the effects on mental health in oncology mental health works, and finally, chapter 7 reviews Covid-19 in Mexico, where there were high numbers of cases as well as deaths due to the virus.

I wish to thank the staff at IntechOpen, especially the Publishing Process Manager, Ms. Dolores Kuzelj, for her excellent support throughout the publication process. I am also grateful to the contributing authors for their excellent chapters.

Dr. Nicolas Padilla-Raygoza
Department of Research and Technological Development,
Directorate of Teaching and Research,
Institute of Public Health from Guanajuato State,
Guanajuato, Mexico

References

[1] Subsecretaría de Prevención y Promoción de la Salud. Secretaría de Salud. Mexico: Informe Técnico Semanal COVID-19; 2022. Available from: https://www.gob.mx/salud/documentos/informe-tecnico-diario-covid19-2022

Section 1

Prevention or Treatment of COVID-19

Chapter 1

Therapeutic Interventions for COVID-19

Martina Smolic, Reham Dawood, Ghada Salum, Mai Abd El Meguid, Moataza Omran and Robert Smolic

Abstract

SARS-CoV-2, a novel coronavirus, is currently represented a major public health concern. The high transmission rate of this virus increases the mortality rate worldwide. To date, significant efforts and restricted regulations were performed around the world to control this crisis effectively, but unfortunately, there is no specific and successful therapy for COVID-19. Many approaches have been repurposed for SARS-CoV-2 treatment such as antivirals and anti-inflammatories. Furthermore, antibody therapies are one of the main and important approaches of SARS-CoV-2 infection treatment. In recent trials, various immunotherapeutic interventions such as convalescent plasma therapy and monoclonal antibodies, as well as immunomodulatory agents are being proposed. However, the development of a vaccine that provides durable protective immunity will be the most effective therapy for controlling possible epidemics of this virus. The current review summarized all the proposed therapeutic approaches together with information on their safety and efficacy in treating COVID-19, as well as the vaccine candidates. The provided comprehensive information regarding the applied therapeutic strategies against COVID-19 might help the scientific community in any progress toward the treatment of COVID-19 infection.

Keywords: SARS-CoV-2-immune response, vaccine, therapeutic interventions, antiviral drugs, immunity

1. Introduction

To date (August 2022), over 600,114,721 have been detected worldwide as positive COVID-19 cases with more than ~6,470,118 deaths in 228 countries [1]. In 2002–2003, the globe was first exposed to coronavirus through severe acute respiratory syndrome (SARS), and in 2011, it was first exposed to middle east respiratory syndrome (MERS) [2]. Then, toward the end of 2019, the current coronavirus (SARS-CoV-2) COVID-19 emerged in Wuhan, China [3]. COVID-19 is a contagious respiratory disease caused by the coronavirus 2 (SARS-CoV-2) that causes severe acute respiratory syndrome [4]. The virus is mostly transmitted by droplets and direct contact [5].

The disease's clinical symptoms are diverse, ranging from asymptomatic to severe illness, up to 20% of symptomatic individuals facing a high risk of mortality [6].

Critical illnesses include acute respiratory distress syndrome, septic shock, coagulopathies, refractory metabolic acidosis, and multi-organ dysfunction [7, 8]. Worse clinical outcomes have been linked to older age, male sex, and comorbidities [9]. To date, the factors associated with the disease severity of COVID-19 have not been clearly identified. It was demonstrated that both viral and host factors are implicated in treatment outcomes [10]. However, the pathogenesis of COVID-19 is closely associated with host factors, particularly cellular immunity in patients [11].

2. Genomics of SARS-CoV-2

SARS-CoV-2, such as other coronaviruses, is an enveloped, single-stranded, and positive-sense RNA virus with a non-segmented genome of 30 kb (**Figure 1**) [12]. The viral genome encodes 16 nonstructural proteins (NSPs) needed for pathogenesis and virus replication, four structural proteins including envelope (E), membrane (M), nucleocapsid (N), and spike (S) glycoproteins, all of which are important for virus genotyping and therapeutic strategies, and nine other accessory genes (**Figure 1**) [13]. There is a huge similarity between the first published SARS-CoV-2 genome and SARS-CoV, especially in the spike protein revealing the high transmission rate from human to human [14].

There is a huge data rising on the viral genomics and its transcriptomic level involving the virus-host protein interactions. These data are highly needed for the drug discovery, vaccine development, and public health strategies.

The ACE2 gene expresses the angiotensin-converting enzyme-2 in several human cells. Several studies reported that the spike protein has a 10–20 times higher affinity for binding to the ACE2 receptor than SARS-CoV, which explains the SARS-CoV-2's higher transmission rate [15].

The host ACE2 receptor is located in abundance on epithelial cells that line the alveoli and bronchioles of the lungs, as well as endothelial cells and myocytes that line the pulmonary blood vessels [16]. The ACE2 gene is also expressed in the small intestine, which could clarify the gastrointestinal symptoms appeared with the viral infection [17].

The spike (S) protein is thought to be the key protein involved in viral entry into target cells [18].

The host transmembrane serine protease 2 (TMPRSS2) "primes" the S protein by cleaving it into two active domains: S1 and S2. The S1 domain can then engage with the ACE2 receptor, while the S2 subunit helps the virus fuse with the target cell, facilitating the viral entry [18]. Blocking the viral entry pathway through ACE2 and TMPRSS2 represents one of the therapeutic strategies that can prevent the virus attachment with the host cell.

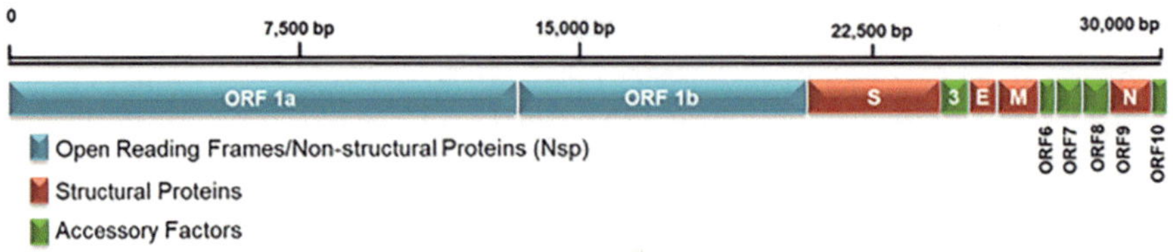

Figure 1.
(a) Illustrative representation of the SARS-CoV-2 genome presenting the location of the structural, nonstructural, and accessory proteins. The figure is created by BioRender program.

3. Mechanism of immune systems in the human body against COVID-19

Both innate and adaptive immunity are required to fight against SARS-CoV-2. The innate immunity includes monocytes, dendritic cells (DCs), granulocytes, and natural killer (NK) cells, while the adaptive immune system includes B and T cells. Severe patients are characterized by the following: Lymphopenia with a drop in CD4+ and CD8+ T cells, lymphocyte activation and dysfunction, an increase in circulating neutrophils with the appearance of circulating neutrophil precursors, and loss of the monocytes function and impaired the function of NK and DCs [19, 20].

Inflammatory cytokine levels are elevated, particularly interleukin-6 and IL-1 [21]. On the other hand, the interferon response is delayed, while the levels of immunoglobulin G (IgG) and total antibodies are increased [22, 23]. Immune disorders, which are characterized by an elevated inflammatory profile, are frequent in severe infections and sepsis and finally ends up with immunosuppression. For severe COVID-19, a similar method has been proposed [24, 25]. Owing to the absence of the effective antiviral therapy, the immunological response of the body is a critical element in disease severity and clinical outcome. Thus, clearer picture regarding the cellular immune response through the disease progression is highly required for establishing diagnostic indicators and potential therapeutic strategies against COVID-19.

During the SARS-CoV-2 infection, the cellular and molecular cascades orchestrate the activation, recruitment, and resolution of the antiviral immune response. These cascades fine-tune the balance between viral eradication and immune injury. Multiple innate immune identification pathways fight viruses during infection [26]. Within the first few hours, The innate immune system inhibits virus replication by releasing type I/III interferon [27], pro-inflammatory cytokines (including: IL-1, IL-6, and IL-18), and chemokines (including: CCL2 and CCL7 and then adaptive immunity is activated.)

Following the SARS-CoV-2 infection, T cells are highly involved in the viral clearance process, whereas humoral immune response is mainly involved in the production of neutralizing antibodies to block the viral entry. T lymphocytes directly attack the infected cells, and they stimulate the cytokines production to boost the immune response of T lymphocytes and other immunocompetent cells such as B lymphocytes and macrophages. To defend the host from nonspecific injury, the body then diminishes innate immunity [28].

Innate immune cells (DCs and macrophages) and adaptive mediated- cell types (regulatory B cells and T cells) establish an inflammation repair status when viruses have been eradicated.

4. Vaccine development

To monitor the global SARS-CoV-2 pandemic, a vaccine development becomes mandatory. The development of a vaccine that provides durable protective immunity will be the most effective therapy for controlling possible epidemics of this virus. The ideal vaccine should be safe, effective, durable, and accessible to a large population. Moreover, the virus genome has the ability to mutate so that it is necessary to develop a safe and pangenotypic vaccine to be effective toward any SARS-CoV-2 variants.

The majority of vaccine approaches have the ability to generate neutralizing antibodies against specific proteins, particularly the spike protein. Some adjuvant components can be added to the vaccine to stimulate the immunity and reduce the amount of antigen required for each vaccine dose. As of August 2022, 222 vaccine candidates were included in the international clinical phase, and 774 vaccines were included in the preclinical phase [29]. The vaccine platforms include viral vector nonreplicating vaccines, protein subunits, DNA-based vaccines, RNA-based vaccines, viral vector replicating vaccines, virus such as particle, live attenuated virus, and bacterial antigen spore expression vector (**Figure 2**) [31, 32].

Several years of research are needed to develop a safe vaccine that can be used in clinical trials. Vaccine evaluation is usually performed in phases after development [33]. Preclinical testing on cell lines and animal models is required in Phase I, followed by testing on a small number of people to affirm immune system stimulation [33]. Phase II involves examining hundreds of people, including children and the elderly, to ensure safety in a new cohort [34]. Finally, thousands of people will be tested in the Phase III trial. During this phases, scientists administer vaccines to volunteers and monitor how many of the placebo and vaccine groups become infected. Typically, these trials are used to monitor if the vaccine provides protection against the virus and detect the absence/presence of adverse effects. Phase III trials are sufficiently large to report efficacy rates, as well as rare side effects.

Of all the vaccines in clinical trials with the SARS-CoV-2 variant, the RNA vaccine appears to be more effective than other vaccines because it requires the development of a large number of vaccines with a limited budget. Although clinical trials are harmless, immune responses elicited by antigens stimulated by RNA vaccines are fewer than those found in animal models [35, 36]. Similar to RNA - based vaccines, DNA-based vaccines are easier and cheaper to provide better safety, efficacy, and long-term immune response. Nevertheless, it has not been approved for human use because it has not elicited a strong enough immune response to be safe. Vaccines based on highly immunogenic vectors, on the other hand, have been shown to induce effective immune responses.

The vaccines that have been registered in phase III clinical trial include vector vaccines (University of Oxford/AstraZeneca, Janssen Pharmaceutical Companies and Gamaleya National Research Centre), mRNA-based vaccines (Pharma/Pfizer and Moderna/National Institute of Allergy and Infectious Diseases), inactivated vaccines (Beijing Institute of Biological Products, Wuhan Institute of Biological Products, and adjuvant recombinant protein nanoparticles (Novavax) [37].

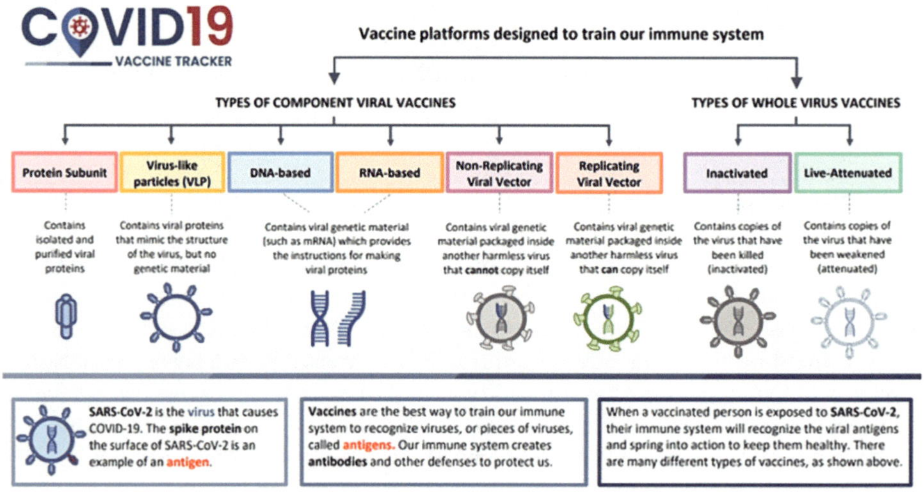

Figure 2.
Illustrates the all the types of approaches for the vaccine development [30].

4.1 Nucleic acid—based vaccine

The nucleic acid vaccine depends on the delivery of the viral genetic codes rather than the viral protein; the transcription and translation processes performed by the host are used to encode the antigen inside the cell before its presentation through the class I of MHC. The technology is relatively new, and no approved nucleic acid vaccines have been used beyond the COVID-19.

4.2 BNT162b2 mRNA COVID-19 vaccine (Pfizer)

BNT162b2 is a lipid nanoparticle–formulated [38], nucleoside-modified RNA expressing the full-length of spike gene, adapted by two proline modifications to keep its structure in the prefusion conformation. Two 30 ug doses of Pfizer vaccine produced significant neutralizing antibody titers directed against SARS-CoV-2, and particular CD8+ and CD4+ T cell responses in healthy individuals in trials done in the United States and Germany [39]. Furthermore, Pfizer vaccine's reactogenicity profile reflected minimal side effects. The development of the BNT162b2 vaccine into phase 3 was encouraged by these findings. The tolerability, safety, immunoreactivity, and efficacy of 30 μg of BNT162b2 in controlling COVID-19 were evaluated in individuals, which are 16 years old or older [40].

4.3 The mRNA-1273 SARS-CoV-2 vaccine (Moderna)

The mRNA1273 vaccine is an mRNA-based lipid nanoparticle encapsulated vaccine expressing the fusion-stabilized full-length spike protein of (SARS-CoV-2) [40]. The moderna vaccine revealed 94.1% efficacy at stopping COVID-19 severity. mRNA-1273's efficacy is comparable to that of the previously disclosed BNT162b2 mRNA vaccination [41].

5. Recombinant vaccines/viral vectors

Viral vector platform involves the insertion of the target gene that encodes for the target protein within an engineered. The viral vector can be able or disabled to replicate there are several viral vectors that are used in the recombinant vaccines such as vesicular stomatitis virus (VSV), adenovirus (Ad), measles virus (MV), alphaviruses, poxviruses, and herpes virus. These types permit the introduction of 5 kb the target gene and have been shown to induce cellular and humoral immunity. The possibility of preexisting immunity to viral vectors, such as Ad5 and MV in vaccine recipients, is one of the major concerns for this platform, which could reduce the vaccine's effectiveness [42]. To avoid this problem, methods such as selecting adenoviral serotypes with low human prevalence (Ad26 or Ad35) have been used.

6. ChAdOx1 nCOVID-19 (AstraZeneca)

A new COVID-19 vaccine is currently in clinical trials; it was developed largely to prevent MERS [43]. This vaccine involves the genetic code of the SARS-CoV-2 spike protein inserted inside an adenovirus vector. The results of the phase 1/2, single-blind, randomized controlled trial revealed that the spike-specific T cell response was detected on day 14, whereas the anti-spike IgG antibodies peaked on day 28. Neutralizing antibodies were generated in 91% of individuals after receiving the first dose and all individuals generated neutralizing antibodies after the booster dose. The safety and immunogenicity results for the ChAdOx1 nCoV-19 candidate vaccine support the entry of this vaccine into phase 3 clinical trials [44].

7. Ad26.COV2.S

The one-shot Ad26.COV2.S vaccine is a recombinant; replication-deficient viral vector denoted human adenovirus type 26 (Ad26) vector expressing the entire sequence of SARS-CoV-2 spike protein in a prefusion-stabilized shape [45, 46]. Other Ad26-based vaccines, such as an authorized Ebola vaccine, have been found to be safe and generate long-lasting immune responses. In preclinical SARS-CoV-2 challenge studies [47, 48], Ad26.COV2.S caused persistent protection at low doses [49], and preliminary clinical data showed that a single dosage of virus particles was safe and elicited sufficient humoral and cellular immune responses [46]. ENSEMBLE trial showed that the vaccine achieved 52.0 and 64.0% efficacy against moderate to severe–critical COVID-19 with onset at least 2 weeks and at least 3 weeks after vaccination, respectively, and achieved 73.1 and 81.7% efficacy against severe–critical COVID-19, respectively [50]. Ad26.COV2.S could be preserved for up to 2 years in a conventional freezer and 3 months in a fridge, making travel, storage, and use in a pandemic much easier.

8. Sputnik V

Gam-COVID-Vac, developed by the Russia's Gamaleya Research Institute of Epidemiology and Microbiology, is composed of two vector vaccines, based on rAd type 26 (rAd26) and rAd type 5 (rAd5)—both of which express the full-length spike protein (rAd26-S and rAd5-S). Both rAd26-S and rAd5-S are injected intramuscularly separately after 3 weeks interval. The results of the phase 1/2 clinical trials revealed the vaccine safety and immunogenicity in the healthy individuals. Therefore, the vaccine was authorized in Russia in accordance with the national laws. In a randomized, controlled phase 3 trial in Russia, including 21,862 participants, they detected the anti-RBD specific IgG titers, neutralizing antibody titers, and cellular immune response. The proposed regimen of vaccination generates both B cell and T cell responses, with 91·6% efficacy against SARS-CoV-2. The vaccine is preserved and dispersed at −18°C but storage at 2–8°C, an optimum temperature for worldwide supply, has also been licensed by the Ministry of Health of the Russian Federation [51].

9. Sputnik light

It is a new single-dose vaccine based on recombinant replication-deficient adenovirus type 26 (rAd26) vector expressing the spike (S) glycoprotein as an attempt to meet the vaccine demand. The "Sputnik Light" single-dose rAd26 vector-based COVID-19 vaccine has a favorable safety profile and generates significant humoral, and cellular immune responses in both seronegative and seropositive subjects [52].

10. CoviShield - Oxford/AstraZeneca vaccine (AZD1222)

Serum Institute of India's COVID-19 vaccine, called Covishield, is a version of the Oxford-AstraZeneca vaccine that manufacturers in India produce locally. (Covishield) has a favorable benefit-risk profile, with remarkable potential to prevent infections and diminish mortality worldwide [53]. It was proved that might protect people from various SARS-CoV-2 variants. The vaccine efficacy is found to be 95% of recipients and stop the disease progression in those infected after vaccination. In phase 3 clinical trial, they demonstrated that the AZD1222 vaccine was tolerable and successful in suppressing clinical symptoms and severe infection across different ethnic groups that recruited older individuals [54].

11. Inactivated vaccine candidate, BBIBP-CorV Sinopharm

Inactivated vaccine development is a well-established platform that is widely adopted for the prevention and control of the virus transmission such as influenza virus and poliovirus. This platform uses the whole organism but inactivated through chemical or physical methods. In this phase 1/2 trial, the BBIBP-CorV inactivated vaccine, given as a two-dose immunization, was safe and well tolerated. The BBIBP-CorV vaccine has the ability to induce humoral immune response in all vaccinated individuals. In preclinical studies, it was observed that the cBBIBP-CorV able to elicit sufficient neutralizing antibody titers in animal model, which have the capacity to protect against SARS-CoV-2 [55]. The generated antibodies against SARS-CoV-2 by the immunization of BBIBP-CorV reached the peak on day 42. The neutralizing antibodies stimulated by BBIBP-CorV have a pangenotypic effect and can prevent multiple SARS-CoV-2 strains infection. These data reveal the BBIBP-CorV has the potential to give cross-protection against different SARS-CoV-2 strains [56].

12. CoronaVac (Sinovac life sciences, Beijing, China)

CoronaVac (Sinovac Life Sciences, Beijing, China) represents one of the inactivated vaccine platform and revealed high immunogenic effects in the preclinical studies in mice, rats, and nonhuman primates. The generated antibodies produced from the immunization of CoronaVac have the ability to neutralize several SARS-CoV-2 variants. Following a SARS-CoV-2 challenge in macaques, the data showed that CoronaVac conferred partial or complete protection and prevent the severe interstitial pneumonia with no detectable antibody-dependent increase of infection, supporting the advance to human clinical trials [57].

The SARS-CoV-2 (CN02 strain) has been transfected into the vero cells and then the virus was collected, treated with β-propiolactone. Then the virus was purified, and absorbed onto aluminum hydroxide. The aluminum hydroxide is used as an adjuvant to induce cellular immunity. The vaccine used in the phase 1 study was prepared using cell factory technology, while the vaccine used in phase2 was prepared by using a highly automated bioreactor. The results showed that the CoronaVac (Sinovac) produced for the phase 2 clinical trial has been enhanced the immunogenic results. Vaccine doses of 3 and 6 μg were injected intramuscularly on either day 0 and day 14 or day 0 and day 28, depending on the cohort. Two doses (days 0 and 28) of 6 μg vaccine yielded the largest antibody recovery, but 3 μg was selected for phase 3 studies based on production capacity (seroconversion rates of 100 and 97%, respectively) [58].

Concerns have been raised about the level of the generated antibodies. The geometric mean titer (GMT) of neutralizing S-IgG was lower than that of convalescent human serum (HCS) while the antibodies arising from natural infection was (mean GMT23.8-65.4). Meanwhile, the results of other vaccine candidates showed that GMT S IgG was superior to HCS. The low immunogenicity of CoronaVac's is represented as one of the obstacles that face this vaccine. The low immunogenic effect of CoronaVac's is may be due to the alteration of S protein induced by the chemical compounds. These vaccine doses were proven to confer the protection against SARS-CoV-2 infection in macaques. CoronaVac is proved to be tolerated and able to generate humoral responses against COVID-19. These findings are paving the way for its emergency use in China and on phase 3 clinical trials. The therapeutic value of CoronaVac remains to be evaluated.

13. Recombinant protein based vaccine (Novavax)

Novavax vaccine is composed of an engineered baculovirus with a modified spike gene. Then the baculovirus transfects the Sf9 moth cell lines, which produce and display the spike protein on their cell membranes. The spike proteins are then extracted and assembled onto a synthetic lipid nanoparticle [59]. Novavax's unique nanoparticle technology used an adjuvants called Matrix-M, to boost immune system and induce high levels of neutralizing antibodies [60]. In Phase 1–2 clinical trial of a Novavax vaccine, the immunological responses produced by NVX-CoV2373 appeared to be higher than those seen in COVID-19 serum [61]. The Matrix-M1 adjuvant elicited CD4+ T cell responses with a Th1 phenotypic bias.

14. Experimental therapeutic interventions

14.1 Convalescent plasma (CP) therapy

Because an effective vaccine and specific antiviral therapies are no longer available, there is a mandatory demand to develop an alternative approach for COVID-19 treatment, particularly in severe patients. For many centuries, convalescent plasma (CP) therapy, a type of adaptive immunotherapy, has been approved to treat a variety of infectious diseases. CP therapy has been used successfully in the treatment of MERS, SARS, and the H1N1 virus with adequate safety and efficacy [62, 63].

Convalescent plasma received from cured COVID-19 patients with generated humoral response directed toward the virus possesses a high concentration of neutralizing antibodies capable of preventing the viral entry and eliminating the virus from blood stream and lung tissues [64]. The first important determining factor in the success of the CP therapy is the neutralizing antibody titer. It was found in a small sample study of MERS-CoV infection that the titer of the neutralizing antibody should be greater than 1:80% to achieve successful CP therapy [63]. Finding suitable donors with high level of neutralizing antibody represents the cornerstone. Cao et al. [65] revealed that the level of neutralizing antibody to SARS-CoV diminished gradually 4 months after the recovery, eventually reaching undetectable levels in 25.6% (total IgG) and 16.1% t (neutralizing antibodies) of patients 36 months later.

According to a study of MERS-CoV infected patients and high risk group, the prevalence of MERS-CoV IgG seroreactivity was estimated to be very low (2.7%), and the antibodies titer decreased rapidly within 3 months [66]. According to these findings, the neutralizing antibodies were a short-lived humoral immune response, and plasma from recently recovered patients should be more effective.

The second key factor that determined the success of treatment is treatment intervention point. The best treatment outcomes were observed in patients with SARS who received CP infusion by day 14 highlighting the necessity of timely rescue therapy. In recent study, they showed that all the transfused patients with neutralizing antibody titer above 1:640 achieved serum SARS-CoV-2 RNA negativity and accompanied with an elevation in lymphocyte counts and oxygen saturation, as well as an improvement in liver function and CRP. The findings suggest that antibodies found in CP alleviated immune system inflammation and overreaction.

Several approaches have been established to isolate and characterize the neutralizing antibodies generated by the convalescent COVID-19 as an attempt to generate effective antibodies as a therapy for COVID-19 [67, 68]. For example, AbCellera, a private Canadian company has developed a human IgG1 monoclonal Abs-based therapeutics for coronavirus infection in collaboration with Eli Lilly. Clinical studies for such antibodies have already been authorized in China.

14.2 Antiviral drugs

Several antiviral drugs have been adopted as potential candidate to treat SARS-CoV-2. The viral life cycle steps can be used as potential drug targets. The viral entry, nonstructural protein, and immune regulation are the promising drug targets **Figure 3**.

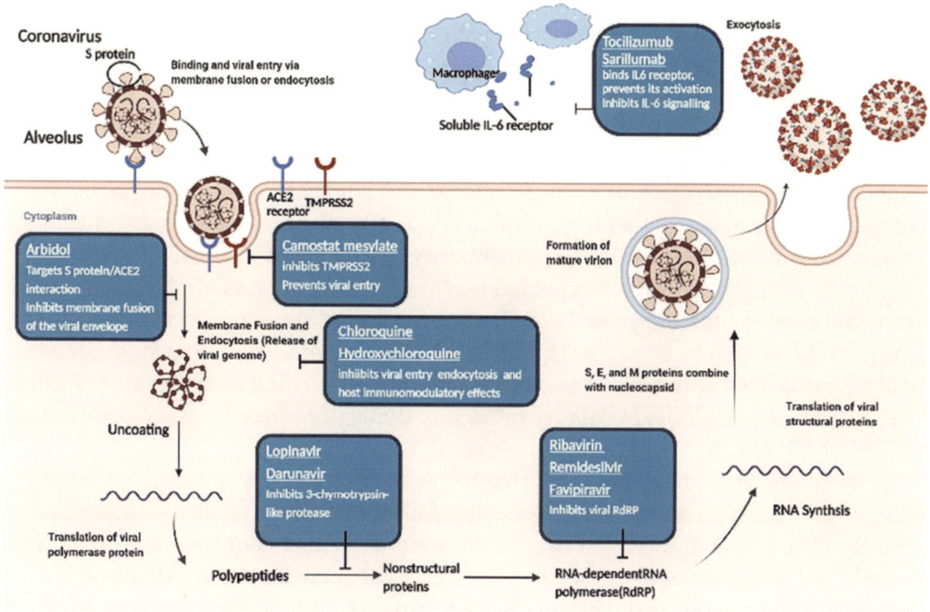

Figure 3.
A diagram represents host immune system stimulated by the virus and viral life cycle within target cells. The figure is created by BioRender program.

14.3 Chloroquine and hydroxychloroquine

Chloroquine and hydroxychloroquine have been permitted for the treatment of malaria and rheumatoid arthritis (RA) and systemic lupus erythematosus (SLE) as they have anti-inflammatory activity. These compounds have the ability to inhibit the virus replication through decreasing the endosomal acidification as SARS-CoV-2 needs the acidic media of the endosome for successful replication [69, 70].

Chloroquine has been shown an antiviral activity against SARS-CoV-2 through *in vitro* study [71]. With the use of chloroquine for the treatment of COVID-19, a clinical trial in China reported efficacy with improved pneumonia severity and an acceptable safety profile [72]. Hydroxychloroquine is a chloroquine derivative that is more stable and has a better clinical safety profile than chloroquine. It also has inhibitory activity toward SARS-CoV-2. When taken in conjunction with azithromycin, it has been proven to provide complete cure and virus clearance in COVID-19 patients [73].

Recent study showed that the combination of azithromycin and hydroxychloroquine has discouraging results in the critically ill SARS-CoV-2 infected patients, which may lead to perform more controlled research before final recommendations for chloroquine/hydroxychloroquine in the treatment of COVID-19 are made [74].

Chloroquine and hydroxychloroquine are zinc ionophores, and zinc has been found to block the activity of coronavirus's RNA-dependent RNA polymerase enzyme [75, 76]. As a result, one reason for some of these clinical trials' limited success might well be the lack of zinc supplementation, which may be required to obtain the medicinal value of these drugs on SARS-CoV-2 and other RNA virus infections [77].

14.4 Lopinavir/ritonavir and other antiretroviral

Lopinavir/Ritonavir is a combined approved drug used for the treatment of HIV. Lopinavir is a protease inhibitor that prevents virus particle maturation, whereas ritonavir sustains the lopinavir's plasma level by inhibiting CYP3A enzymes, which delays lopinavir's breakdown in the liver [78]. The data obtained from *in vitro*, and animal studies revealed its potential inhibitory effect against SARS-CoV, MERS, and SARS-CoV-2 [78, 79]. For COVID-19 therapy, lopinavir-ritonavir has been administered alone or in combination with alpha interferon or chloroquine/hydroxychloroquine with modest effectiveness [80, 81]. However, contradictory results have been released from China regarding impact of COVID-19 patients who are very unwell [82]. Recently, a randomized study of 199 hospitalized patients with COVID-19 who were treated with lopinavir/ritonavir reported no significant change in viral load, duration of hospital stay, or mortality rate [82]. The study was too small to conclude the potential role of lopinavir/ritonavir on the COVID-19 treatment and experts suggested that further randomized clinical trial to be conducted to confirm or deny the lack of effect.

As a result, more clinical trials are needed to determine the success of this therapy for COVID-19, which is now being conducted.

Furthermore, it has been observed that patients who received lopinavir/ritonavir regimen have had gastrointestinal adverse side includes diarrhea, nausea, and hepatotoxicity [83]. Elevated level of transaminases was commonly noticed in COVID-19 infected patients as one of the side effects, the case that may be worsened by any viral coinfection and/or combined therapy [84]. Recently RCT found that around half of lopinavir/ritonavir patients suffered a lot of unfavorable side effects, and around sixth of patients stopped medication owing to gastrointestinal complications [82]. Elevated transaminases triggered by drugs have special concern since it has the potential to worsen COVID-19-induced liver impairment. Notably, the elevation of liver enzyme is an undesired criterion in numerous COVID-19 research study, suggesting that lopinavir/ritonavir triggered liver toxicity may restrict patients' access to those medications [85].

Darunavir/cobicistat (DRV/c) is a protease inhibitor used for the treatment for HIV. *In vitro* study demonstrated an antiviral activity of darunavir against SARS-CoV-2.

In a randomized controlled clinical trial aimed to monitor the efficacy of DRV in treating COVID-19 patients, the obtained results failed to show a significant benefit of using (DRV/c) therapy beyond the standard care in the mild COVID-19 infected patients [86]. In this regard, HIV1 protease inhibitors may not exhibit clinically significant activity against SARS-CoV-2.

14.5 Favipiravir (Favilavir or Avigan)

Favipiravir (FPV) is a safe and effective RNA polymerase inhibitor developed in Japan for different RNA viral infection including influenza [87, 88]. The antiviral activity of the FPV against SARS-CoV-2 has been approved in a controlled study conducted in China [89]. Through the COVID-19 patients' medication, the effects of FPV vs. LPV/RTV were examined in this study. The FPV-treated individuals showed a considerably superior therapeutic response, with rapid viral clearance and a higher amelioration in chest radiography. Upon these hopeful data, the FPV therapy has been authorized as first anti-COVID-19 medication by the Chinese National Medical Products Administration [68].

14.6 Remdesivir (GS-5734)

Remdesivir is a nucleotide analog compound that inhibits the viral RNA-dependent RNA polymerase; its inhibitory effect against MERS CoV, SARS-CoV, and SARS-CoV-2 replication has been confirmed in *in vitro* studies and in animal models [90, 91]. The development company (Gilead Sciences, USA) declared a clinical improvement in more than half of patients (36 of 53) [92]. However, recent study in China did not exhibit significant clinical benefit, with the exception of the diminishment in the time required for recovery [93]. Additionally, in some patients, treatment with remdesivir had to be stopped prematurely due to unfavorable complications in 12% of patients compared to 5% of patients receiving placebo. Similar results were also reported in the first clinical trial in the United States. Repeated clinical trials of remdesivir in multiple countries must be performed to obtain more convincing recommendations for use in COVID-19 patients. Moreover, the efficacy of remdesivir against the novel COVID-19 variants are not well evaluated and the acquired drug resistance to the mutant strains should be monitored.

15. Immunomodulatory agents

Several data pointed out the role of immunosuppressive treatments (e.g., corticosteroids, inhibitors, IL-6 inhibitors, interleukin (IL)-1 inhibitors, and kinase inhibitors) and immunomodulators (e.g., interferon alpha and beta (IFNα), (IFNβ), in COVID-19. The rationale for using these immunomodulatory/immunosuppressive agents for the treatment of COVID-19 is the involvement of the pro-inflammatory mediator with pieces of evidence of cytokine release storm (i.e., critical hyper inflammation and immune imbalance), which is required to induce multi-organ dysfunction and failure, worsening COVID-19 prognosis [94].

The humanized monoclonal antibody (tocilizumab) has been developed to bind with the receptor of IL-6 (IL-6R) that has been licensed by the FDA for the treatment of RA, giant cell arteritis, and systemic juvenile idiopathic arthritis [95]. IL-6 was involved in the production of cytokine storm (CS) found in ICU-admitted COVID-19 patients [95]. As a result, it has been offered as a possible treatment for such individuals [96]. Tocilizumab, for example, has been approved to be used as an immunosuppressive agent in severely ill COVID-19 patients in China and Italy, with promising findings [97, 98]. In a Chinese cohort, the administration of tocilizumab showed an improvement in patients with severe symptoms. While in the Italian cohort, the administration of tocilizumab in a COVID-19 patient with pneumonia revealed good alterations in CT findings within 14 days of therapy [99]. It is proving to be a viable treatment for treating. Several randomized controlled trials (NCT04310228, ChiCTR200002976) of tocilizumab alone or in combination in COVID-19 patients with severe pneumonia are ongoing in China and are included in the current Chinese protocol for the treatment of COVID-19 patients [100].

Sarilumab, another IL6 receptor antagonist approved for the treatment of R, is being investigated in a phase 2/3 clinical trial in hospitalized patients with severe COVID-19 (NCT04315298) [101].

Bevacizumab is monoclonal antibodies directed against vascular endothelial growth factor that are undergoing clinical trials in China and the United States NCT04275414).

Interferon alpha and beta have been studied against nCoV, and interferon beta is active against MERS [102, 103]. The use of interferon for the treatment of SARS-CoV-2 cannot be recommended at this time because of contradictory *in vitro* and animal results and the lack of clinical trials [104]. Current Chinese regulations recommend interferon as an alternative to combination therapy.

16. Soluble human (ACE2)

For successful COVID-19 treatment, it has been proposed that blocking the interaction between the viral spike protein and ACE2, which is the host receptor for SARS-CoV-2 infection, might be a viable treatment [105].

This finding has opened debate about whether ACE inhibitors and/or angiotensin receptor blockers could be used to treat COVID-19 or, conversely, aggravate the disease [106]. ACE inhibitors can cause a decrease in angiotensin I levels, triggering a possible negative feedback loop, which in turn activates more ACE2 receptors to interact with available angiotensin I substrates. On the contrary, angiotensin receptor blockers may theoretically provide clinical benefit by blocking the ACE2 receptor. There are inconsistent *in vitro* results to verify if these drugs are harmful or protective in patients with COVID-19. There is insufficient data to conclude that patients on long-term ACE inhibitors, or ARB medication are at a higher risk of poor COVID-19 outcomes [107].

A recent *in vitro* investigation found that humanized recombinant soluble ACE2 (hrsACE2) may inhibit SARS-CoV-2 replication, resulting in significantly lower virus load in vero cell lines in a dose-dependent manner [108]. These findings are encouraging because they offer up a new avenue for using hrsACE2 to prevent SARS-CoV-2 infection at an early stage by inhibiting the virus's entrance into target cells, potentially saving patients from lung damage.

17. Umifenovir (also known as arbidol)

Umifenovir (also known as arbidol) is a potent antiviral drug with a novel mechanism that inhibits viral envelope fusion by targeting the S protein/ACE2 interaction [109]. Based on *in vitro* studies demonstrating action against SARS, the medication is now authorized in Russia and China for the treatment and prevention of influenza. It is also gaining interest in treating COVID-19 [110]. The current influenza treatment dosage of 200 mg orally every 8 hours is being investigated for COVID-19 therapy (NCT04260594). In China, only limited clinical experience with umifenovir for COVID-19 has been reported. In a non-randomized analysis of 67 COVID-19 patients, therapy with umifenovir for 9 days was related with reduced fatality rates and higher discharge rates than patients who did not get the drug [111]. This finding cannot approve the success of umifenovir for COVID-19 treatment, but several RCTs are required for further investigation of this agent.

18. Corticosteroids

Corticosteroids are used to reduce the host's inflammatory process in the lungs, which can contribute to acute lung damage and acute respiratory distress syndrome (ARDS). COVID-19 induces severe endothelial and alveolar damage as a result of host-mediated excessive inflammation and cytokine storm [7]. Excessive inflammation and an unregulated immunological response are the major causes of COVID-19-related death [112]. Corticosteroids are extensively used and well tolerated over the world. They have the potential to minimize the risk of cytokine storms and inflammation in COVID-19 [113]. They may also be able to control the course of respiratory failure and mortality by regulating inflammation-mediated lung damage [113, 114]. Previous research regarding the efficacy of corticosteroid therapy in severe pneumonia [115] revealed a link between corticosteroid usage and a lower risk of ARDS, as well as shorter hospital stay duration [116]. However, corticosteroids have the potential to greatly reduce the use of mechanical ventilation required in COVID-19 patients while also limiting major side effects. Additionally, for individuals with COVID-19, a pulse dosage of methylprednisolone for fewer than 7 days may be a useful therapy strategy [117].

However, side effects such as delayed virus clearance and an increased risk of subsequent infection may balance this advantage. In an observational study, no link has been found between corticosteroids and high survival rate in patients with SARS and MERS but reported a link between delayed virus clearance and high incidence of comorbidities such as hyperglycemia, psychosis, and avascular necrosis [102, 118]. Moreover, a meta-analysis of 10 observational studies of 6548 patients with influenza pneumonia in 2019 found that corticosteroids were linked to an increased risk of death and twice the risk of secondary infection [119]. While the effectiveness of corticosteroids in ARDS and septic shock is generally controversial, Russell and colleagues [120] claimed that individuals with bacterial infection are more likely to benefit from corticosteroids than those with viral infections. The data currently supports the use of corticosteroids in COVID-19 patients; however, additional study is needed on the type, dose, start time, and duration.

19. The situation in Egypt and the governmental efforts to control the COVID-19 transmission

Here in the next few lines, we summarize the situation of COVID-19 statistics in Egypt and focus on the efforts and actions of the Egyptian government to regulate and halt the COVID-19 transmission.

To date (August 2022), over 515,198 confirmed laboratory cases have been detected with more than ~24,786 deaths in Egypt, according to the official website of the Egyptian MOH (https://www.care.Gov.eg/Egypt Care/index.aspx accessed August, 2022).

The decreased incidence of COVID-19 in Egypt does not match the reality. The recorded number of the infected cases depended only on the laboratory-confirmed cases; however, many Egyptians have been infected with SARS-CoV-2 and have been homelily isolated till recovery without performing the COVID-19 test. The decreased incidence in Egypt may be related to the large population, minimal screening testing, warmth and humidity, and use of the bacille Calmette-Guerin (BCG) vaccination. Host genetic alteration has also been shown to influence indigenous Africans' resistance to a range of infectious diseases [121]. The appearance of SARS-CoV-2 strains are raising high public health problem owing to their high transmission rate, higher pathogenicity, and in some cases, ability to infect vaccinated people (vaccine breakthrough). The risk of death is increased significantly with age [122, 123] and

Antipyretic	Paracetamol
Cough suppressants	Acelylcysteine
Anticoagulants	Enoxaparine
Fluid therapy	According to the condition of the patient
Multivitamins	Vitamin C or Zinc
Antiviral drugs and Antibiotics	Hydroxychloroquine - Ivermectin – Favipiravir - Remdesivir - Lopinavir/Ritonavir - Monoclonal antibodies - Convalescent plasma - Azithromycin - Nitazoxanide- Oseltamivir - Ribavirin - Interferon beta 1b - Doxycycline
Anti-inflammatory	Hydrocortisone – Dexamethasone - Methylprednisolone
Supplement	Lactoferrin
Immunosuppressive	Tocilizumab
Oxygen therapy	
Mechanical ventilation	

For patients with COVID-19, the Egyptian Ministry of Health approved a standard of a care treatment strategy that included
By the end of May 2020, the Egyptian MOH guideline recommended that mild and some moderate cases will be managed by home isolation

Figure 4.
The protocol for the treatment of COVID-19 patients approved by the MOH [126].

comorbidities (cardiovascular disease, cancer, diabetes, and chronic lung disease) [6, 124]. Patients with one or more comorbidities had low survival rates [125].

The Egyptian Ministry of Health and Population (MOH) has built a hotline service to help persons in need of medical advice. The Egyptian government has launched a huge disinfection program using chlorine-containing disinfectants as lipid solvents that targeted all squares, workplaces, and touristic spots. The standard of care treatment strategy for COVID-19 patients has been approved by the Egyptian Ministry of Health (**Figure 4**) [127]. The Egyptian Ministry of Health has advised that mild and possibly moderate cases can be handled at home.

Egypt has been receiving nine approved anti-COVID-19 vaccines since December 2020 including Moderna (mRNA-1273), Pfizer/BioNTech(BNT162b2), Gamaleya (Sputnik Light), Janssen (Johnson & Johnson): (Ad26.COV2.S), Sinovac(CoronaVac), Sinopharm (BBIBP-CorV), AstraZeneca vaccine, and Sputnik V. Priority categories for vaccination include (A) health care workers in quarantine, fever, and chest hospitals, (B) immunocompromised patients, and the elderly, and (C) eventually all people over the age of 18. Egypt has begun the distribution of COVID-19 vaccines as of March 2021. It was estimated that the percentage of fully vaccinated individual is 19.8% while the percentage with at least one dose is 31.8% [128]. In developing countries, the application of strict regulations to halt the viral transmission is difficult due to human overpopulation, so it is mandatory to highlight the importance of boosting the host immunity.

20. Conclusion

COVID-19 patients are characterized by lymphopenia and elevated cytokine levels, which could be used as indicators for disease progression. COVID-19 has immunological profiles that can lead to microbial infection and various organ failures. As a result, improving lymphopenia and decreasing inflammation may be helpful therapeutic methods for COVID-19 patients. Currently, antiviral drugs and immunotherapies are two principal therapeutic approaches for COVID-19, whereas vaccines are still considered the most effective strategy to get rid of this virus. COVID-19 vaccine advancements are encouraging because this is the first time vaccine development has moved so quickly. Vaccinology-based research advances have assured that the most crucial public health intervention is created in a timely manner. Researchers and clinicians still need to perform better planned controlled clinical trials and collect more biological samples to better understand host immune responses to pathogens and their implications for the treatment of patients.

Author details

Martina Smolic[1*], Reham Dawood[2], Ghada Salum[2], Mai Abd El Meguid[2], Moataza Omran[2] and Robert Smolic[3]

1 Faculty of Dental Medicine and Health Osijek, Department of Pharmacology and Biochemistry, J.J. Strossmayer University of Osijek, Osijek, Croatia

2 Department of Microbial Biotechnology, Biotechnology Research Institute, National Research Centre, Giza, Egypt

3 Faculty of Medicine Osijek, Department of Pharmacology, Josip Juraj Strossmayer University of Osijek, Osijek, Croatia

*Address all correspondence to: msmolic@fdmz.hr

IntechOpen

© 2023 The Author(s). Licensee IntechOpen. This chapter is distributed under the terms of the Creative Commons Attribution License (http://creativecommons.org/licenses/by/3.0), which permits unrestricted use, distribution, and reproduction in any medium, provided the original work is properly cited.

References

[1] World Health Organization. WHO Coronavirus Disease (COVID-19) Dashboard. 2021. Available from: https:// covid19.who.int/

[2] Prompetchara E, Ketloy C, Palaga T. Immune responses in COVID-19 and potential vaccines: Lessons learned from SARS and MERS epidemic. Asian Pacific Journal of Allergy and Immunology. 2020;**38**(1):1-9

[3] Li Q, Guan X, Wu P, Wang X, Zhou L, Tong Y, et al. Early transmission dynamics in Wuhan, China, of novel coronavirus–infected pneumonia. New England Journal of Medicine. 2020;**382**(13):1199-1207

[4] Xu X, Chen P, Wang J, Feng J, Zhou H, Li X, et al. Evolution of the novel coronavirus from the ongoing Wuhan outbreak and modeling of its spike protein for risk of human transmission. Science China Life sciences. 2020;**63**(3): 457-460. Epub 2020/02/06. DOI: 10.1007/ s11427-020-1637-5

[5] Chu DK, Duda S, Solo K, Yaacoub S, Schunemann H. Physical Distancing, Face masks, and eye protection to prevent person-to-person transmission of SARS-CoV-2 and COVID-19: A systematic review and meta-analysis. Journal of Vascular Surgery. 2020;**72**(4):1500. Epub 09/21. doi: 10.1016/j.jvs.2020.07.040

[6] Huang C, Wang Y, Li X, Ren L, Zhao J, Hu Y, et al. Clinical features of patients infected with 2019 novel coronavirus in Wuhan, China. Lancet. 2020;**395**(10223):497-506. Epub 2020/01/28. DOI: 10.1016/ s0140-6736(20)30183-5

[7] Wiersinga WJ, Rhodes A, Cheng AC, Peacock SJ, Prescott HC. Pathophysiology, transmission, diagnosis, and treatment of coronavirus disease 2019 (COVID-19): A review. Journal of the American Medical Association. 2020;**324**(8):782-793. DOI: 10.1001/jama.2020.12839

[8] Tian D, Ye Q. Hepatic complications of COVID-19 and its treatment. Journal of Medical Virology. 2020;**92**(10):1818-1824. DOI: 10.1002/jmv.26036

[9] Guan W-j, Ni Z-y, Hu Y, Liang W-h, Ou C-q, He J-x, et al. Clinical characteristics of coronavirus disease 2019 in China. New England Journal of Medicine. 2020;**382**(18):1708-1720. DOI: 10.1056/NEJMoa2002032

[10] Zhang X, Tan Y, Ling Y, Lu G, Liu F, Yi Z, et al. Viral and host factors related to the clinical outcome of COVID-19. Nature. 2020;**583**(7816):437-440. Epub 2020/05/21. DOI: 10.1038/ s41586-020-2355-0

[11] Rydyznski Moderbacher C, Ramirez SI, Dan JM, Grifoni A, Hastie KM, Weiskopf D, et al. Antigen-specific adaptive immunity to SARS-CoV-2 in acute COVID-19 and associations with age and disease severity. Cell. 2020;**183**(4):996-1012 e19. DOI: 10.1016/j.cell.2020.09.038

[12] Andersen KG, Rambaut A, Lipkin WI, Holmes EC, Garry RF. The proximal origin of SARS-CoV-2. Nature Medicine. 2020;**26**(4):450-452. DOI: 10.1038/s41591-020-0820-9

[13] Kim D, Lee JY, Yang JS, Kim JW, Kim VN, Chang H. The architecture of SARS-CoV-2 transcriptome. Cell. 2020;**181**(4):914-21 e10. DOI: 10.1016/j. cell.2020.04.011

[14] Zhu N, Zhang D, Wang W, Li X, Yang B, Song J, et al. A novel coronavirus

from patients with pneumonia in China, 2019. New England Journal of Medicine. 2020;**382**(8):727-733. DOI: 10.1056/NEJMoa2001017

[15] Luan J, Lu Y, Jin X, Zhang L. Spike protein recognition of mammalian ACE2 predicts the host range and an optimized ACE2 for SARS-CoV-2 infection. Biochemical and Biophysical Research Communications. 2020;**526**(1):165-169. DOI: 10.1016/j.bbrc.2020.03.047

[16] Hamming I, Timens W, Bulthuis M, Lely A, Navis G, van Goor H. Tissue distribution of ACE2 protein, the functional receptor for SARS coronavirus. A first step in understanding SARS pathogenesis. The Journal of Pathology. 2004;**203**(2):631-637. DOI: 10.1002/path.1570

[17] Ong SWX, Tan YK, Chia PY, Lee TH, Ng OT, Wong MSY, et al. Air, surface environmental, and personal protective equipment contamination by severe acute respiratory syndrome coronavirus 2 (SARS-CoV-2) from a symptomatic patient. Journal of the American Medical Association. 2020;**323**(16):1610-1612. DOI: 10.1001/jama.2020.3227

[18] Hoffmann M, Kleine-Weber H, Schroeder S, Kruger N, Herrler T, Erichsen S, et al. SARS-CoV-2 cell entry depends on ACE2 and TMPRSS2 and is blocked by a clinically proven protease inhibitor. Cell. 2020;**181**(2):271-80 e8. DOI: 10.1016/j.cell.2020.02.052

[19] Schultze JL, Aschenbrenner AC. COVID-19 and the human innate immune system. Cell. 2021;**184**(7):1671-1692. Epub 2021/03/21. DOI: 10.1016/j.cell.2021.02.029

[20] Sette A, Crotty S. Adaptive immunity to SARS-CoV-2 and COVID-19. Cell. 2021;**184**(4):861-880. Epub 2021/01/27. DOI: 10.1016/j.cell.2021.01.007

[21] Ye Q, Wang B, Mao J. The pathogenesis and treatment of the `cytokine Storm' in COVID-19. The Journal of Infection. 2020;**80**(6):607-613. Epub 2020/04/14. DOI: 10.1016/j.jinf.2020.03.037

[22] Chen G, Wu D, Guo W, Cao Y, Huang D, Wang H, et al. Clinical and immunological features of severe and moderate coronavirus disease 2019. The Journal of Clinical Investigation. 2020;**130**(5):2620-2629. DOI: 10.1172/JCI137244

[23] Giamarellos-Bourboulis EJ, Netea MG, Rovina N, Akinosoglou K, Antoniadou A, Antonakos N, et al. Complex immune dysregulation in COVID-19 patients with severe respiratory failure. Cell Host & Microbe. 2020;**27**(6):992-1000. e3. DOI: 10.1016/j.chom.2020.04.009

[24] Remy KE, Brakenridge SC, Francois B, Daix T, Deutschman CS, Monneret G, et al. Immunotherapies for COVID-19: Lessons learned from sepsis. The Lancet Respiratory Medicine. 2020;**8**(10):946-949. DOI: 10.1016/S2213-2600(20)30217-4

[25] Ritchie AI, Singanayagam A. Immunosuppression for hyperinflammation in COVID-19: A double-edged sword? Lancet. 2020;**395**(10230):1111. DOI: 10.1016/S0140-6736(20)30691-7

[26] Koch J, Steinle A, Watzl C, Mandelboim O. Activating natural cytotoxicity receptors of natural killer cells in cancer and infection. Trends in Immunology. 2013;**34**(4):182-191. DOI: 10.1016/j.it.2013.01.003

[27] Stetson DB, Medzhitov R. Type I interferons in host defense. Immunity. 2006;**25**(3):373-381. DOI: 10.1016/j.immuni.2006.08.007

[28] Dong Kim K, Zhao J, Auh S, Yang X, Du P, Tang H, et al. Adaptive immune cells temper initial innate responses. Nature Medicine. 2007;**13**(10):1248-1252. DOI: 10.1038/nm1633

[29] Jha AK, Kumar R, Goenka MK, Dayal VM. Emerging treatment and prevention strategies against COVID-19: A brief update. Journal of Digestive Endoscopy. 2020;**11**(1):69-72. Epub 05/16. DOI: 10.1055/s-0040-1712547

[30] COVID-19 Vaccine Tracker. TYPES OF VACCINES. Available from: https://covid19.trackvaccines.org/types-of-vaccines/ [Accessed: December 2, 2022].

[31] Abboud H, Zheng C, Kar I, Chen CK, Sau C, Serra A. Current and emerging therapeutics for neuromyelitis optica spectrum disorder: Relevance to the COVID-19 pandemic. Multiple Sclerosis and Related Disorders. 2020;**44**:102249. Epub 2020/06/12. DOI: 10.1016/j.msard.2020.102249

[32] Yu J, Tostanoski LH, Peter L, Mercado NB, McMahan K, Mahrokhian SH, et al. DNA vaccine protection against SARS-CoV-2 in rhesus macaques. Science. 2020;**369**(6505):806-811. Epub 2020/05/22. DOI: 10.1126/science.abc6284

[33] Merante D. SARS-CoV-2, from its current highly contagious spreading toward the global development of an effective and safe vaccine: Challenges and uncertainties. Expert Opinion on Drug Safety. 2020;**19**(7):771-774. Epub 06/08. DOI: 10.1080/14740338.2020.1773789

[34] Locht C. Vaccines against COVID-19. Anaesthesia, Critical Care & Pain Medicine. 2020;**39**(6):703-705. Epub 2020/10/24. DOI: 10.1016/j.accpm.2020.10.006

[35] Zhang C, Maruggi G, Shan H, Li J. Advances in mRNA vaccines for infectious diseases. Frontiers in Immunology. 2019;**10**(594):594. DOI: 10.3389/fimmu.2019.00594

[36] Prete M, Favoino E, Catacchio G, Racanelli V, Perosa F. SARS-CoV-2 inflammatory syndrome. Clinical features and rationale for immunological treatment. International Journal of Molecular Sciences. 2020;**21**(9). Epub 2020/05/14:3377. DOI: 10.3390/ijms21093377

[37] Tregoning JS, Brown ES, Cheeseman HM, Flight KE, Higham SL, Lemm NM, et al. Vaccines for COVID-19. Clinical and Experimental Immunology. 2020;**202**(2):162-192. Epub 2020/09/17. DOI: 10.1111/cei.13517

[38] Pardi N, Tuyishime S, Muramatsu H, Kariko K, Mui BL, Tam YK, et al. Expression kinetics of nucleoside-modified mRNA delivered in lipid nanoparticles to mice by various routes. Journal of Controlled Release. 2015;**217**:345-351

[39] Sahin U, Muik A, Vogler I, Derhovanessian E, Kranz LM, Vormehr M, et al. BNT162b2 induces SARS-CoV-2-neutralising antibodies and T cells in humans. Nature. 2020;**595**(7868):572-577

[40] Polack FP, Thomas SJ, Kitchin N, Absalon J, Gurtman A, Lockhart S, et al. Safety and efficacy of the BNT162b2 mRNA Covid-19 vaccine. New England Journal of Medicine. 2020;**383**(27):2603-2615. DOI: 10.1056/NEJMoa2034577

[41] Dickerman BA, Gerlovin H, Madenci AL, Kurgansky KE, Ferolito BR, Figueroa Muñiz MJ, et al. Comparative effectiveness of BNT162b2 and mRNA-1273 vaccines in U.S. veterans. New England Journal of Medicine. 2021;**386**:105-115. DOI: 10.1056/NEJMoa2115463

[42] Rauch S, Jasny E, Schmidt KE, Petsch B. New vaccine technologies to combat outbreak situations. Frontiers in Immunology. 2018;**9**:1963. Epub 2018/10/05. DOI: 10.3389/fimmu.2018.01963

[43] van Doremalen N, Haddock E, Feldmann F, Meade-White K, Bushmaker T, Fischer RJ, et al. A single dose of ChAdOx1 MERS provides protective immunity in rhesus macaques. Science Advances. 2020;**6**(24):eaba8399

[44] Folegatti PM, Ewer KJ, Aley PK, Angus B, Becker S, Belij-Rammerstorfer S, et al. Safety and immunogenicity of the ChAdOx1 nCoV-19 vaccine against SARS-CoV-2: A preliminary report of a phase 1/2, single-blind, randomised controlled trial. Lancet. 2020;**396**(10249):467-478. DOI: 10.1016/S0140-6736(20)31604-4

[45] Bos R, Rutten L, van der Lubbe JE, Bakkers MJ, Hardenberg G, Wegmann F, et al. Ad26 vector-based COVID-19 vaccine encoding a prefusion-stabilized SARS-CoV-2 spike immunogen induces potent humoral and cellular immune responses. npj Vaccines. 2020;**5**(1):1-11

[46] Sadoff J, Le Gars M, Shukarev G, Heerwegh D, Truyers C, de Groot AM, et al. Interim results of a phase 1-2a trial of Ad26. COV2. S Covid-19 vaccine. New England Journal of Medicine. 2021;**384**(19):1824-1835

[47] Salisch NC, Stephenson KE, Williams K, Cox F, van der Fits L, Heerwegh D, et al. A double-blind, randomized, placebo-controlled phase 1 study of Ad26. ZIKV. 001, an Ad26-vectored anti–Zika virus vaccine. Annals of Internal Medicine. 2021;**174**(5):585-594

[48] Williams K, Bastian AR, Feldman RA, Omoruyi E, de Paepe E, Hendriks J, et al. Phase 1 safety and immunogenicity study of a respiratory syncytial virus vaccine with an adenovirus 26 vector encoding prefusion F (Ad26. RSV. preF) in adults aged≥ 60 years. The Journal of Infectious Diseases. 2020;**222**(6):979-988

[49] Mercado NB, Zahn R, Wegmann F, Loos C, Chandrashekar A, Yu J, et al. Single-shot Ad26 vaccine protects against SARS-CoV-2 in rhesus macaques. Nature. 2020;**586**(7830):583-588

[50] Sadoff J, Gray G, Vandebosch A, Cárdenas V, Shukarev G, Grinsztejn B, et al. Safety and efficacy of single-dose Ad26.COV2.S vaccine against Covid-19. New England Journal of Medicine. 2021;**384**(23):2187-2201. DOI: 10.1056/NEJMoa2101544

[51] Logunov DY, Dolzhikova IV, Shcheblyakov DV, Tukhvatulin AI, Zubkova OV, Dzharullaeva AS, et al. Safety and efficacy of an rAd26 and rAd5 vector-based heterologous prime-boost COVID-19 vaccine: An interim analysis of a randomised controlled phase 3 trial in Russia. Lancet. 2021;**397**(10275):671-681. Epub 2021/02/06. DOI: 10.1016/s0140-6736(21)00234-8

[52] Tukhvatulin AI, Dolzhikova IV, Shcheblyakov DV, Zubkova OV, Dzharullaeva AS, Kovyrshina AV, et al. An open, non-randomised, phase 1/2 trial on the safety, tolerability, and immunogenicity of single-dose vaccine "sputnik light" for prevention of coronavirus infection in healthy adults. The Lancet Regional Health – Europe. 2021;**11**:100241. DOI: 10.1016/j.lanepe.2021.100241

[53] Health Canada. AstraZeneca/Covishield COVID-19 Vaccine: What you Should Know. Health Canada; 26 February 2021. Archived from the original on 20 April 2021 [Accessed: March 26, 2021]

[54] Sharun K, Singh R, Dhama K. Oxford-AstraZeneca COVID-19 vaccine (AZD1222) is ideal for resource-constrained low- and middle-income countries. Annals of Medicine and Surgery (Lond). May 2021;**65**:102264. DOI: 10.1016/j.amsu.2021.102264. Epub 2021 Mar 31. PMID: 33815783; PMCID: PMC8010342

[55] Wang H, Zhang Y, Huang B, Deng W, Quan Y, Wang W, et al. Development of an inactivated vaccine candidate, BBIBP-CorV, with potent protection against SARS-CoV-2. Cell. 2020;**182**(3):713-21.e9

[56] Xia S, Zhang Y, Wang Y, Wang H, Yang Y, Gao GF, et al. Safety and immunogenicity of an inactivated SARS-CoV-2 vaccine, BBIBP-CorV: A randomised, double-blind, placebo-controlled, phase 1/2 trial. The Lancet Infectious Diseases. 2021;**21**(1):39-51. Epub 10/15. DOI: 10.1016/S1473-3099(20)30831-8

[57] Gao Q, Bao L, Mao H, Wang L, Xu K, Yang M, et al. Development of an inactivated vaccine candidate for SARS-CoV-2. Science. 2020;**369**(6499):77-81

[58] Zhang Y, Zeng G, Pan H, Li C, Hu Y, Chu K, et al. Safety, tolerability, and immunogenicity of an inactivated SARS-CoV-2 vaccine in healthy adults aged 18-59 years: A randomised, double-blind, placebo-controlled, phase 1/2 clinical trial. The Lancet Infectious Diseases. 2021;**21**(2):181-192. DOI: 10.1016/S1473-3099(20)30843-4

[59] Tian J-H, Patel N, Haupt R, Zhou H, Weston S, Hammond H, et al. SARS-CoV-2 spike glycoprotein vaccine candidate NVX-CoV2373 immunogenicity in baboons and protection in mice. Nature Communications. 2021;**12**(1):1-14

[60] Bengtsson KL, Song H, Stertman L, Liu Y, Flyer DC, Massare MJ, et al. Matrix-M adjuvant enhances antibody, cellular and protective immune responses of a Zaire Ebola/Makona virus glycoprotein (GP) nanoparticle vaccine in mice. Vaccine. 2016;**34**(16):1927-1935

[61] Keech C, Albert G, Cho I, Robertson A, Reed P, Neal S, et al. Phase 1-2 trial of a SARS-CoV-2 recombinant spike protein nanoparticle vaccine. New England Journal of Medicine. 2020;**383**(24):2320-2332. DOI: 10.1056/NEJMoa2026920

[62] Cheng Y, Wong R, Soo YO, Wong WS, Lee CK, Ng MH, et al. Use of convalescent plasma therapy in SARS patients in Hong Kong. European Journal of Clinical Microbiology & Infectious Diseases. 2005;**24**(1):44-46. Epub 2004/12/24. DOI: 10.1007/s10096-004-1271-9

[63] Ko JH, Seok H, Cho SY, Ha YE, Baek JY, Kim SH, et al. Challenges of convalescent plasma infusion therapy in Middle East respiratory coronavirus infection: A single Centre experience. Antiviral Therapy. 2018;**23**(7):617-622. Epub 2018/06/21. DOI: 10.3851/imp3243

[64] Marano G, Vaglio S, Pupella S, Facco G, Catalano L, Liumbruno GM, et al. Convalescent plasma: New evidence for an old therapeutic tool? Blood Transfusion. 2016;**14**(2):152-157. Epub 2015/12/18. DOI: 10.2450/2015.0131-15

[65] Cao WC, Liu W, Zhang PH, Zhang F, Richardus JH. Disappearance of antibodies to SARS-associated coronavirus after recovery. The New England Journal of Medicine. 2007;**357**(11):1162-1163. Epub 2007/09/15. DOI: 10.1056/NEJMc070348

[66] Arabi YM, Hajeer AH, Luke T, Raviprakash K, Balkhy H, Johani S, et al. Feasibility of using convalescent plasma immunotherapy for MERS-CoV

infection, Saudi Arabia. Emerging Infectious Diseases. 2016;**22**(9):1554-1561. Epub 2016/08/18. DOI: 10.3201/eid2209.151164

[67] Hodgson J. The pandemic pipeline. Nature Biotechnology. 2020;**38**(5):523-532. DOI: 10.1038/d41587-020-00005-z

[68] Tu Y-F, Chien C-S, Yarmishyn AA, Lin Y-Y, Luo Y-H, Lin Y-T, et al. A review of SARS-CoV-2 and the ongoing clinical trials. International Journal of Molecular Sciences. 2020;**21**(7):2657. DOI: 10.3390/ijms21072657

[69] Akpovwa H. Chloroquine could be used for the treatment of filoviral infections and other viral infections that emerge or emerged from viruses requiring an acidic pH for infectivity. Cell Biochemistry and Function. 2016;**34**(4):191-196. DOI: 10.1002/cbf.3182

[70] Li C, Zhu X, Ji X, Quanquin N, Deng YQ, Tian M, et al. Chloroquine, a FDA-approved drug, prevents Zika virus infection and its associated congenital microcephaly in mice. eBioMedicine. 2017;**24**:189-194. DOI: 10.1016/j.ebiom.2017.09.034

[71] Wang M, Cao R, Zhang L, Yang X, Liu J, Xu M, et al. Remdesivir and chloroquine effectively inhibit the recently emerged novel coronavirus (2019-nCoV) in vitro. Cell Research. 2020;**30**(3):269-271. Epub 2020/02/06. DOI: 10.1038/s41422-020-0282-0

[72] Gao J, Tian Z, Yang X. Breakthrough: Chloroquine phosphate has shown apparent efficacy in treatment of COVID-19 associated pneumonia in clinical studies. BioScience Trends. 2020;**14**(1):72-73. DOI: 10.5582/bst.2020.01047

[73] Gautret P, Lagier JC, Parola P, Hoang VT, Meddeb L, Mailhe M, et al. Hydroxychloroquine and azithromycin as a treatment of COVID-19: Results of an open-label non-randomized clinical trial. International Journal of Antimicrobial Agents. 2020;**56**(1):105949. Epub 2020/03/25. DOI: 10.1016/j.ijantimicag.2020.105949

[74] Molina JM, Delaugerre C, Le Goff J, Mela-Lima B, Ponscarme D, Goldwirt L, et al. No evidence of rapid antiviral clearance or clinical benefit with the combination of hydroxychloroquine and azithromycin in patients with severe COVID-19 infection. Medecine et maladies infectieuses. 2020;**50**(4):384. Epub 2020/04/03. DOI: 10.1016/j.medmal.2020.03.006

[75] Kaushik N, Subramani C, Anang S, Muthumohan R, Shalimar NB, et al. Zinc salts block hepatitis E virus replication by inhibiting the activity of viral RNA-dependent RNA polymerase. Journal of Virology. 2017;**91**(21):e00754-e00717. DOI: 10.1128/JVI.00754-17

[76] Liang SH, Southon AG, Fraser BH, Krause-Heuer AM, Zhang B, Shoup TM, et al. Novel fluorinated 8-Hydroxyquinoline based metal Ionophores for exploring the metal hypothesis of Alzheimer's disease. ACS Medicinal Chemistry Letters. 2015;**6**(9):1025-1029. DOI: 10.1021/acsmedchemlett.5b00281

[77] Shittu MO, Afolami OI. Improving the efficacy of chloroquine and Hydroxychloroquine against SARS-CoV-2 may require zinc additives - a better synergy for future COVID-19 clinical trials. Le infezioni in medicina. 2020;**28**(2):192-197 Epub 2020/04/27

[78] Wilde AH, Jochmans D, Posthuma CC, Zevenhoven-Dobbe JC, Nieuwkoop SV, Bestebroer TM, et al. Screening of an FDA-approved compound library identifies four

small-molecule inhibitors of Middle East respiratory syndrome coronavirus replication in cell culture. Antimicrobial Agents and Chemotherapy. 2014;**58**(8):4875-4884. DOI: 10.1128/AAC.03011-14

[79] Chu CM, Cheng VCC, Hung IFN, Wong MML, Chan KH, Chan KS, et al. Role of lopinavir/ritonavir in the treatment of SARS: Initial virological and clinical findings. Thorax. 2004;**59**(3):252-256. DOI: 10.1136/thorax.2003.012658

[80] Lim J, Jeon S, Shin HY, Kim MJ, Seong YM, Lee WJ, et al. Case of the index patient who caused tertiary transmission of COVID-19 infection in Korea: The application of Lopinavir/ritonavir for the treatment of COVID-19 infected pneumonia monitored by quantitative RT-PCR. Journal of Korean Medical Science. 2020;**35**(6):e79. Epub 2020/02/15. DOI: 10.3346/jkms.2020.35.e79

[81] Yan D, Liu X-Y, Zhu Y-N, Huang L, Dan B-T, Zhang G-J, et al. Factors associated with prolonged viral shedding and impact of Lopinavir/ritonavir treatment in patients with SARS-CoV-2 infection. European Respiratory Journal. 2020;**56**(1):2000799. DOI: 10.1101/2020.03.22.20040832

[82] Cao B, Wang Y, Wen D, Liu W, Wang J, Fan G, et al. A trial of Lopinavir–ritonavir in adults hospitalized with severe Covid-19. New England Journal of Medicine. 2020;**382**(19):1787-1799. DOI: 10.1056/NEJMoa2001282

[83] Vecchio G, Zapico V, Catanzariti A, Carboni Bisso I, Las HM. Adverse effects of lopinavir/ritonavir in critically ill patients with COVID-19. Medicina. 2020;**80**(5):439-441 Epub 2020/10/14

[84] Wu C, Chen X, Cai Y, Xia J, Zhou X, Xu S, et al. Risk factors associated with acute respiratory distress syndrome and death in patients with coronavirus disease 2019 pneumonia in Wuhan, China. JAMA Internal Medicine. 2020;**180**(7):934-943. Epub 2020/03/14. DOI: 10.1001/jamainternmed.2020.0994

[85] ClinicalTrials.gov. Available from: https://clinicaltrials.gov/ [Accessed: March 18, 2020]

[86] Chen J, Xia L, Liu L, Xu Q, Ling Y, Huang D, et al. Antiviral activity and safety of Darunavir/Cobicistat for the treatment of COVID-19. Open Forum Infectious Diseases. 2020;**7**(7):ofaa241. Epub 2020/07/17. DOI: 10.1093/ofid/ofaa241

[87] Furuta Y, Komeno T, Nakamura T. Favipiravir (T-705), a broad spectrum inhibitor of viral RNA polymerase. Proceedings of the Japan Academy Series B, Physical and biological sciences. 2017;**93**(7):449-463. Epub 2017/08/05. DOI: 10.2183/pjab.93.027

[88] Smee DF, Tarbet EB, Furuta Y, Morrey JD, Barnard DL. Synergistic combinations of favipiravir and oseltamivir against wild-type pandemic and oseltamivir-resistant influenza a virus infections in mice. Future Virology. 2013;**8**(11):1085-1094. Epub 2014/02/25. DOI: 10.2217/fvl.13.98

[89] Cai Q, Yang M, Liu D, Chen J, Shu D, Xia J, et al. Experimental treatment with Favipiravir for COVID-19: An open-label control study. Engineering. 2020;**6**(10):1192-1198. DOI: 10.1016/j.eng.2020.03.007

[90] Sheahan TP, Sims AC, Graham RL, Menachery VD, Gralinski LE, Case JB, et al. Broad-spectrum antiviral GS-5734 inhibits both epidemic and zoonotic coronaviruses. Science Translational Medicine. 2017;**9**(396):eaal3653. DOI: 10.1126/scitranslmed.aal3653

[91] de Wit E, Feldmann F, Cronin J, Jordan R, Okumura A, Thomas T, et al. Prophylactic and therapeutic remdesivir (GS-5734) treatment in the rhesus macaque model of MERS-CoV infection. Proceedings of the National Academy of Sciences. 2020;**117**(12):6771-6776. DOI: 10.1073/pnas.1922083117

[92] Grein J, Ohmagari N, Shin D, Diaz G, Asperges E, Castagna A, et al. Compassionate use of Remdesivir for patients with severe Covid-19. New England Journal of Medicine. 2020;**382**(24):2327-2336. DOI: 10.1056/NEJMoa2007016

[93] Wang Y, Zhang D, Du G, Du R, Zhao J, Jin Y, et al. Remdesivir in adults with severe COVID-19: A randomised, double-blind, placebo-controlled, multicentre trial. Lancet. 2020;**395**(10236):1569-1578. DOI: 10.1016/S0140-6736(20)31022-9

[94] Fajgenbaum DC, June CH. Cytokine Storm. The New England Journal of Medicine. 2020;**383**(23):2255-2273. Epub 2020/12/03. DOI: 10.1056/NEJMra2026131

[95] Zhang S, Li L, Shen A, Chen Y, Qi Z. Rational use of Tocilizumab in the treatment of novel coronavirus pneumonia. Clinical Drug Investigation. 2020;**40**(6):511-518. DOI: 10.1007/s40261-020-00917-3

[96] Ortiz-Martínez Y. Tocilizumab: A new opportunity in the possible therapeutic arsenal against COVID-19. Travel Medicine and Infectious Disease. 2020;**37**:101678. DOI: 10.1016/j.tmaid.2020.101678

[97] Zhang C, Wu Z, Li J-W, Zhao H, Wang G-Q. Cytokine release syndrome in severe COVID-19: Interleukin-6 receptor antagonist tocilizumab may be the key to reduce mortality. International Journal of Antimicrobial Agents. 2020;**55**(5):105954. DOI: 10.1016/j.ijantimicag.2020.105954

[98] Zhao M. Cytokine storm and immunomodulatory therapy in COVID-19: Role of chloroquine and anti-IL-6 monoclonal antibodies. International Journal of Antimicrobial Agents. 2020;**55**(6):105982. DOI: 10.1016/j.ijantimicag.2020.105982

[99] Cellina M, Orsi M, Bombaci F, Sala M, Marino P, Oliva G. Favorable changes of CT findings in a patient with COVID-19 pneumonia after treatment with tocilizumab. Diagnostic and Interventional Imaging. 2020;**101**(5):323-324. DOI: 10.1016/j.diii.2020.03.010

[100] National Health Commission and State Administration of Traditional Chinese Medicine. Diagnosis and treatment protocol for novel coronavirus pneumonia. Available from: https://www.chinalawtranslate.com/wp-content/uploads/2020/03/Who-translation.pdf [Accessed: March 18, 2020]

[101] Sanofi. Sanofi and Regeneron begin global Kevzara (sarilumab) clinical trial program in patients with severe COVID-19 [news release]. 2020. Available from: http://www.news.sanofi.us/2020-03-16-Sanofi-and-Regeneron-begin-global-Kevzara-R-sarilumabclinical-trial-program-in-patients-with-severe-COVID-19 [Accessed: March 18, 2020]

[102] Stockman LJ, Bellamy R, Garner P. SARS: Systematic review of treatment effects. PLoS Medicine. 2006;**3**(9):e343. DOI: 10.1371/journal.pmed.0030343

[103] Morra ME, Van Thanh L, Kamel MG, Ghazy AA, Altibi AMA, Dat LM, et al. Clinical outcomes of current medical approaches for Middle

East respiratory syndrome: A systematic review and meta-analysis. Reviews in Medical Virology. 2018;**28**(3):e1977. DOI: 10.1002/rmv.1977

[104] Totura AL, Bavari S. Broad-spectrum coronavirus antiviral drug discovery. Expert Opinion on Drug Discovery. 2019;**14**(4):397-412. DOI: 10.1080/17460441.2019.1581171

[105] Zhang H, Penninger JM, Li Y, Zhong N, Slutsky AS. Angiotensin-converting enzyme 2 (ACE2) as a SARS-CoV-2 receptor: Molecular mechanisms and potential therapeutic target. Intensive Care Medicine. 2020;**46**(4):586-590. Epub 2020/03/04. DOI: 10.1007/s00134-020-05985-9

[106] Gurwitz D. Angiotensin receptor blockers as tentative SARS-CoV-2 therapeutics. Drug Development Research. 2020;**81**(5):537-540. DOI: 10.1002/ddr.21656

[107] American Heart Association. Patients taking angiotensin converting enzyme inhibitors (ACE-i) or angiotensin receptor blocker (ARB) medications should continue therapy as prescribed [news release]. Published March 17, 2020. Available from: https://newsroom.heart.org/news/patients-taking-ace-i-and-arbs-who-contractcovid-19-should-continue-treatment-unlessotherwise-advised-by-their-physician [Accessed: March 18, 2020]

[108] Monteil V, Kwon H, Prado P, Hagelkruys A, Wimmer RA, Stahl M, et al. Inhibition of SARS-CoV-2 infections in engineered human tissues using clinical-grade soluble human ACE2. Cell. 2020;**181**(4):905-13 e7. DOI: 10.1016/j.cell.2020.04.004

[109] Kadam RU, Wilson IA. Structural basis of influenza virus fusion inhibition by the antiviral drug Arbidol. Proceedings of the National Academy of Sciences. 2017;**114**(2):206-214. DOI: 10.1073/pnas.1617020114

[110] Khamitov RA, Loginova S, Shchukina VN, Borisevich SV, Maksimov VA, Shuster AM. Antiviral activity of arbidol and its derivatives against the pathogen of severe acute respiratory syndrome in the cell cultures. Voprosy Virusologii. 2008;**53**(4):9-13 Epub 2008/09/02

[111] Wang Z, Yang B, Li Q, Wen L, Zhang R. Clinical features of 69 cases with coronavirus disease 2019 in Wuhan, China. Clinical Infectious Diseases. 2020;**71**(15):769-777. DOI: 10.1093/cid/ciaa272

[112] Rowaiye AB, Okpalefe OA, Onuh Adejoke O, Ogidigo JO, Hannah Oladipo O, Ogu AC, et al. Attenuating the effects of novel COVID-19 (SARS-CoV-2) infection-induced cytokine storm and the implications. Journal of Inflammation Research. 2021;**14**:1487-1510. Epub 2021/04/24. DOI: 10.2147/jir.s301784

[113] Bhaskar S, Sinha A, Banach M, Mittoo S, Weissert R, Kass JS, et al. Cytokine storm in COVID-19-Immunopathological mechanisms, clinical considerations, and therapeutic approaches: The REPROGRAM consortium position paper. Frontiers in Immunology. 2020;**11**:1648. Epub 2020/08/06. DOI: 10.3389/fimmu.2020.01648

[114] Horby P, Lim WS, Emberson JR, Mafham M, Bell JL, Linsell L, et al. Dexamethasone in hospitalized patients with Covid-19. The New England Journal of Medicine. 2021;**384**(8):693-704. Epub 2020/07/18. DOI: 10.1056/NEJMoa2021436

[115] Wan YD, Sun TW, Liu ZQ, Zhang SG, Wang LX, Kan QC. Efficacy

and safety of corticosteroids for community-acquired pneumonia: A systematic review and meta-analysis. Chest. 2016;**149**(1):209-219. Epub 2015/10/27. DOI: 10.1378/chest.15-1733

[116] Lu X, Han W, Gao Y-X, Guo S-G, Yu S-Y, Yu X-Z, et al. Efficacy and safety of corticosteroids in immunocompetent patients with septic shock. World Journal of Emergency Medicine. 2021;**12**(2):124-130. DOI: 10.5847/wjem.j.1920-8642.2021.02.007

[117] Cui Y, Sun Y, Sun J, Liang H, Ding X, Sun X, et al. Efficacy and safety of corticosteroid use in coronavirus disease 2019 (COVID-19): A systematic review and meta-analysis. Infectious Diseases and Therapy. 2021;**10**(4):2447-2463. Epub 2021/08/15. DOI: 10.1007/s40121-021-00518-3

[118] Arabi YM, Mandourah Y, Al-Hameed F, Sindi AA, Almekhlafi GA, Hussein MA, et al. Corticosteroid therapy for critically ill patients with Middle East respiratory syndrome. American Journal of Respiratory and Critical Care Medicine. 2017;**197**(6):757-767. DOI: 10.1164/rccm.201706-1172OC

[119] Ni Y-N, Chen G, Sun J, Liang B-M, Liang Z-A. The effect of corticosteroids on mortality of patients with influenza pneumonia: A systematic review and meta-analysis. Critical Care. 2019;**23**(1):99. DOI: 10.1186/s13054-019-2395-8

[120] Russell CD, Millar JE, Baillie JK. Clinical evidence does not support corticosteroid treatment for 2019-nCoV lung injury. Lancet. 2020;**395**(10223):473-475. DOI: 10.1016/S0140-6736(20)30317-2

[121] Gomez F, Hirbo J, Tishkoff SA. Genetic variation and adaptation in Africa: Implications for human evolution and disease. Cold Spring Harbor Perspectives in Biology. 2014;**6**(7):a008524. Epub 2014/07/06. DOI: 10.1101/cshperspect.a008524

[122] Ghweil AA, Hassan MH, Khodeary A, Mohamed AO, Mohammed HM, Abdelazez AA, et al. Characteristics, outcomes and indicators of severity for COVID-19 among sample of ESNA quarantine Hospital's patients, Egypt: A retrospective study. Infection and Drug Resistance. 2020;**13**:2375-2383. DOI: 10.2147/IDR.S263489

[123] Davies NG, Klepac P, Liu Y, Prem K, Jit M, group CC-w, et al. Age-dependent effects in the transmission and control of COVID-19 epidemics. Nature Medicine. 2020;**26**(8):1205-1211. DOI: 10.1038/s41591-020-0962-9

[124] Ergönül Ö, Akyol M, Tanrıöver C, Tiemeier H, Petersen E, Petrosillo N, et al. National case fatality rates of the COVID-19 pandemic. Clinical Microbiology and Infection. 2021;**27**(1):118-124. Epub 2020/09/27. DOI: 10.1016/j.cmi.2020.09.024

[125] Albadawy RM, Jadoon BA, Mogahed MM, Ibrahim ME, Essawy TS, Amin AMA, et al. The impact of comorbidities on the outcomes of Egyptian COVID-19 patients: A follow-up study. Journal of Environmental and Public Health. 2021;**2021**:6662476. Epub 2021/07/10. DOI: 10.1155/2021/6662476

[126] Saied AA, Metwally AA, Madkhali NAB, Haque S, Dhama K. Egypt's COVID-19 recent happenings and perspectives: A mini-review. Frontiers in Public Health. 2021;**9**:696082. DOI: 10.3389/fpubh.2021.696082

[127] Abd El Ghaffar MM, Salem MR, Al Soda MF, Abd El Razik MS, Tahoon MH, Tahoon MF, et al. COVID-19 Pandemic

Preparedness in Egypt's Teaching Hospitals: A Needs Assessment Study. Frontiers in Public Health. 17 Jan 2022;**9**:748666. DOI: 10.3389/fpubh.2021.748666. PMID: 35111710; PMCID: PMC8801519

[128] COVID19 Vaccine Tracker. 9 Vaccines Approved for Use in Egypt. Available from: https://covid19.trackvaccines.org/country/egypt/ [Accessed: January 7, 2022]

Section 2

Complications of COVID-19 in Children

Chapter 2

Multisystem Inflammatory Syndrome in Children (MIS-C)

Felipe Yagnam Rojas

Abstract

The burden of disease caused by the new SARS-CoV-2 coronavirus is focused on adults. In children, this infection manifests as a mild and even asymptomatic acute respiratory illness. Reports in April 2020 described a multisystem inflammatory syndrome in children (MIS-C) occurring 2 to 6 weeks after SARS-CoV-2 wave peak. Clinical manifestations included fever, gastrointestinal symptoms, Kawasaki Disease criteria, hypercoagulability, and laboratory parameters within severe inflammatory range. There is no certainty of the pathophysiology of this syndrome. It is thought to be driven by a post-viral dysregulated immune response. The disease can be life threatening, frequently presented as rapid-onset severe organ failure and need for pediatric critical care support. Cardiovascular dysfunction and coronary involvement are the most serious complications. The clinical and laboratory features of MIS-C indicate that the inflammation is exceptionally high; thus, empirical immunomodulation is the current therapy, leading to good clinical results. Once vaccination against SARS-CoV-2 began, a drop in the incidence of MIS-C happened. In the post-COVID era, permanent vaccination of the population in countries that are already vaccinated is necessary to keep MIS-C incidence rates low. While SARS-CoV-2 is circulating in the world, MIS-C will remain as a differential diagnosis in the evaluation of sick children.

Keywords: children, COVID-19, inflammatory, pediatric, SARS-CoV-2

1. Introduction

The infection caused by the new coronavirus SARS-CoV-2 spread rapidly in the world. At the beginning of 2020, the year in which the disease was declared a pandemic by the World Health Organization (WHO) there was no certainty of its behavior in the adult population, even less how it would affect the children [1]. Time showed that COVID-19 mainly affects adults with fast-spreading lung disease, high rates of hospitalization by respiratory failure secondary to severe pneumonia, and with significant morbidity and mortality [2]. The massive need for medical care caused emergency rooms and hospitalizations around the world to collapse, yet the reality of childhood population at that time was very different. In children, COVID-19 presented as a mild and rare disease, often asymptomatic, with low need for hospitalization and low mortality [3]. Due to this opposite behavior between children and adults and the collapse of health systems around the world, many pediatric services and pediatric intensive care units had to change their care and transform into adult units. These seriously ill adults were treated by staff usually dedicated to child care [4]. Many hypotheses tried to explain this phenomenon in which children were less susceptible to getting sick. No theory seemed to explain by itself the disease opposite behavior between children and adults, but the only clear thing is that infants seemed to cope very well with COVID-19. This is until April 2020, when a series of reports from the United Kingdom and Italy reported the presence of a childhood disease with a clinical presentation similar to Kawasaki Disease or Toxic Shock Syndrome, but temporarily associated with an infection by SARS-CoV-2 [5, 6]. It was a syndrome of generalized inflammation with skin and mucous membrane involvement, which could potentially seriously compromise children. The disease was soon described in the rest of Europe, America, and then around the world. It was called Multisystem Inflammatory Syndrome in children associated with COVID-19 (MIS-C) or Pediatric Inflammatory Multisystem Syndrome (PIMS). Clinical and laboratory criteria were developed to have suspicion and early diagnosis. These recommendations were initially published by WHO and the Centers of Disease Control and Prevention (CDC) and then massified by countless guidelines of pediatric scientific societies and health services throughout the world [7, 8]. The syndrome occurred with severity in a small group of children, even requiring critical care support and connection to mechanical ventilation. It was a diagnostic and therapeutic challenge for pediatric critical care teams, since the severity of these patients was determined by a multisystem compromise of uncertain behavior and not by severe pneumonia as had been seen so far in adults infected with SARS-COV-2. We know now that MIS-C is rare and has low mortality. Although critical care is required in a small group of pediatric patients, the evolution is favorable if the diagnosis and immunomodulatory treatment is instituted in time, with complete recovery of organ involvement in most affected children [9]. The fall in the incidence of COVID-19, as well as the lower severity and decrease in mortality, was the consequence of the massive vaccination in both adults and children. This allowed the viral circulation to decrease, resulting in less SARS-CoV-2 infection in children and therefore a lower incidence of MIS-C [10]. MIS-C is rare; however, it is a differential diagnosis that should be taken into account in pediatric patients, while there is circulation of SARS-CoV-2 in the world. This diagnostic suspicion should be greater in any country with temporary peaks of infection and mainly in countries with low vaccination rates where high viral circulation can cause an increase in the presence of new variants. The SARS-CoV-2 virus is here to stay and consequently, the multisystemic inflammatory response of children to this infection is a real possibility as long as there is viral circulation.

2. Epidemiology

MIS-C is a rare complication of pediatric COVID-19. It is described in <1 percent of children with confirmed SARS-CoV-2 infection [9]. Reports from the United States describe an incidence of 2 per 100,000 infected with COVID-19 under 21 years of age [11]. Despite these reports, the incidence of MIS-C can vary significantly depending on the infectious waves as well as the susceptibility of the population that is directly related to vaccination rates [12, 13]. It mainly affects children over 5 years of age. More than 70% of affected children have no associated comorbidities [14, 15].

It is described more frequently in some races (black, Hispanic, Latino); however, there may be biases influenced by their sociocultural reality [16]. The epidemiology of MIS-C differs from adult SARS-CoV-2 infection. Although most infected children have, like adults, asymptomatic or mild respiratory symptoms, it is in the severe presentation when a difference occurs, presenting as multisystem inflammation and not as severe pneumonia. Children, massively asymptomatic, could act as a reservoir and vector of viral infection, perpetuating the circulation of the new coronavirus in adults, favoring peaks of infection in them [17]. It is these peaks that affect the incidence of MIS-C, which has a temporal association with them. MIS-C appears a few weeks after the peak of SARS-COV2 infection. It is described between 2 and 8 weeks after the population infectious peaks, which means that MIS-C could correspond to an immune-mediated post-infectious disease. The emergence of SARS-COV2 variants has had an impact on the current occurrence of MIS-C. The Omicron wave is described as less severe in adults and with a lower incidence of MIS-C, which was reported worldwide. The Omicron waves showed that the pediatric population that was not fully vaccinated still decreased the incidence of MIS-C [18–22]. The impact of vaccination appears to influence not only the variant, but also the age at which MIS-C occurs, showing an epidemiological change with age shifting to younger children (< 5 years) who are not vaccinated [23, 24]. It is likely that this current decrease in the incidence of MIS-C is multifactorial, being related to the increasing exposure of the population to SARS-COV2, the lower viral circulation, and the massive adult and child vaccination, which probably generates variants with less possibility to create a hyperinflammation syndrome, maintaining the susceptibility of presenting the syndrome to populations with low vaccination rates.

3. Pathophysiology

MIS-C is presented late in relation to the peak of SARS-CoV-2 cases, which is why it is suggested from the outset that it would be an immune-mediated post-infectious disease. The presence of antibodies to SARS-CoV-2 often without a positive PCR made this theory more accurate. Serology is positive even up to 90% of cases; however, the molecular detection of the virus by PCR varies between 20 and 40%. Until now, the exact pathophysiology is unknown, but there are theories that try to explain how SARS-CoV-2 causes such a dysregulated response in children [25].

3.1 Immune dysregulation

SARS-CoV-2 infection in pediatric population would produce a functional activation of phagocytes and complement mediated by immunoglobulin G (IGG), similar to the response of adults with moderate COVID-19, and different to severe adult COVID-19 infection that is primarily mediated by IGA and neutrophils [26]. Once the acute infection has passed, often asymptomatic, the child persists with high levels of IGG similar to acute infection levels and with the ability to activate the immune system later. In addition, the prolonged permanence of the virus in the intestine of children is described. If intestinal inflammation is persistent, the possibility of increased permeability is real, with consequent leakage of viruses into circulation [27]. Single-cell RNA sequencing of peripheral blood mononuclear cells from children with acute MIS-C has been studied, showing low viral and bacterial signatures, suggesting that there are no viral or bacterial infections as triggers of MIS-C [28]. The response of children to the Spike glycoprotein (S) is strong in IGG but weak in immunoglobulin M (IGM). They also have a poor immune response to the nucleocapsid protein (N) [29–31]. Adults on the other hand have a better response to protein S in any types of immunoglobulin, as well as better neutralizing capacity [32]. The asymptomatic nature of the disease in children could be related to this type of immune response. The immunoglobulin response in children with MIS-C is shown in **Figure 1**. Between 20 and 50% of people without exposure to SARS-CoV-2 have T cell reactivity against the virus. This may be due to some cross-reaction between CD4+ T cells and the seasonal coronavirus before the pandemic [33, 34]. Seasonal coronavirus antibodies do not vary between children with MIS-C and children hospitalized for other reasons so the role played by these previously activated T cells in the pathophysiology of MIS-C is not yet clarified [35]. High IFNy levels correlate with high levels of plasma-soluble markers from natural killer (NK) cells and T cells, suggesting that there is an increase in cytotoxic gene expression, which could contribute to tissue damage [28]. There is activation of CD8+ T cells that express inflammatory molecules of the vascular endothelium that could be related to cardiovascular alterations, D-dimer production, thrombocytopenia, and vasoactive drug requirement. This activation would be only in pediatric patients infected with SARS-CoV-2 who develop MIS-C and is related to cytotoxicity although to a less than NK. The proportion of CD8+ T cells decreases as the child's clinical condition improves [28, 36]. Non-specific B cell activation and elevation of plasmablast can be observed [37]. Complement activation is part of the inflammatory process in MIS-C. The elevation of C5b-9 in sick patients is related to endothelial dysfunction. There is an associated within complement activation and thrombotic microangiopathy. Patients with MIS-C have a higher incidence of thrombotic events compared to healthy children or patient COVID-19 without MIS-C [38].

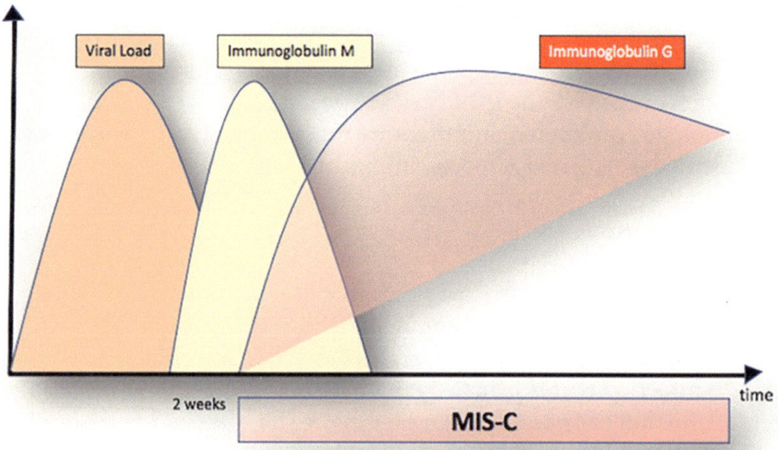

Adapted from Sharma et al. Multisystem inflammatory syndrome in children and Kawasaki disease: a critical comparison. Nat Rev Rheumatol 17, 731–748 (2021).

Immunoglobin M (IGM) is elevated approximately 2 weeks after the peak viral load of SARS-CoV-2. Once the peak of IGM is achieved, the rise of immunoglobulin G (IGG) begins. IGG remains high while IGM falls until it disappears. This period of the time is when multisystemic inflammatory syndrome in children (MIS-C) rise.

Figure 1.
The immunoglobulin response in children with MIS-C.

3.2 Superantigen theory

The virus binds to the immune cell *via* toll-like receptor (TLR) and is endocytosed. A fragment of SARS-CoV-2 spike glycoprotein 1 (S1) is similar to staphylococcal enterotoxin B [39]. This viral structure interacts with a high affinity between the major histocompatibility complex II (MHC II) and CD4+ T cell receptors (TCR). This interaction between MHCII and TCR would be the same that occurs with enterotoxin B of staphylococcus, acting as a superantigen in the pathophysiology of toxic shock syndrome (TSS) [39]. An expansion of TCR β variable gene 11–2 (TRBV11–2) has been found. This TCR correlates with MIS-C severity and serum cytokine levels and it has been associated with HLA class I alleles [40]. Proteins would act as superantigen interacting not only with TCR, but also at the endothelial level between Major Histocompatibility Complex I (MHC I) and CD28+ T cells [41]. The cytokine storm that occurs in TSS occurs during acute staphylococcal infection, whereas in MIS-C SARS-CoV-2 is usually no longer detected, so the superantigen properties of SARS-CoV-2 and its role in the pathophysiology of MIS-C have yet to be confirmed.

3.3 Genetic susceptibility

All pediatric patients infected with SARS-CoV-2 have a similar antibody response, independent of whether they develop MIS-C. The fact that MIS-C only occurs in a small group of children suggests that the immune response is associated with a genetic predisposition. It is thought that there are mutations or polymorphisms of genes that encode molecules that trigger immune cascades, among other TLRs and Fcγ receptors [42]. It has been described that there could be an alteration in genes that regulate the suppression of cytokine signals (SOCS1). An alteration in these genes would mean an impossibility of stopping the inflammatory cascade in these children. Despite all the descriptions seen above, there is no specific genetic alteration that can explain why some children develop MIS-C and other does not.

3.4 Inflammatory mediators

There is an elevation of interleukin (IL) 1B, IL6, IL8, IL10, IL 17A, IFNy, and a series of chemokines that are present in MIS-C and not in pediatric respiratory infection by COVID-19 [43, 44]. E-selectin is a molecular marker of endothelial cell inflammation and is at high levels in children with MIS-C, so endothelial involvement seems to be a contributor to the inflammatory process of all systems [28]. When measuring inflammatory markers, they differ between patients, probably by genetic susceptibility, severity of the disease, and geographic location [25]. The heterogeneity of inflammatory markers does not allow attributing the disease to a single inflammatory pathway.

In summary, MIS-C is due to a post-infectious immune dysregulation and virus-induced cytopathic effects and inflammation in multiple organ systems. Aberrant immune activation may occur by: particular variants of SARS-CoV-2; genetic predisposition (variants in the genes that encode Fcγ receptors, components of the signaling cascades, mutations in genes such as SOCS1 that regulate the immune response); SARS-CoV-2 spike protein and the formation of a superantigen; dysregulated activation of lymphocytes, with production of IGG; and complement activation and autoantibody-mediated endothelial damage (**Figure 2**).

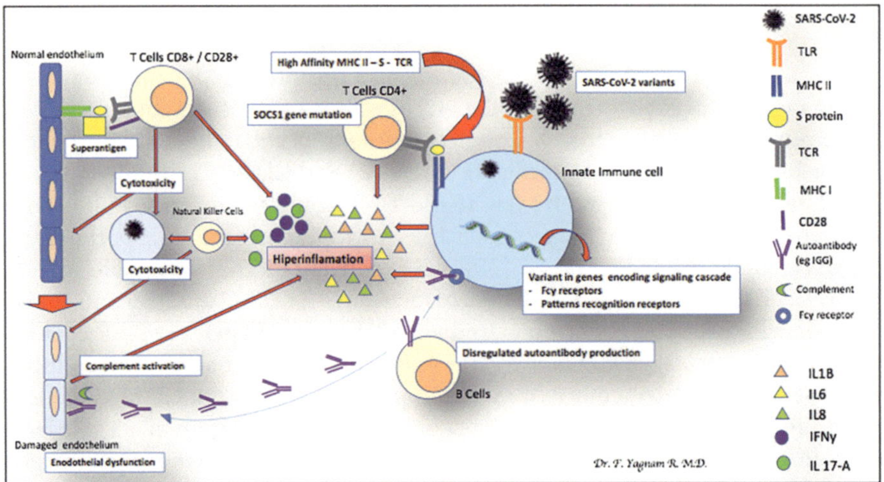

Adapted from Sharma et al. Multisystem inflammatory syndrome in children and Kawasaki disease: a critical comparison. Nat Rev Rheumatol 17, 731–748 (2021).

The immune response could depend on SARS-CoV-2 factors such as the different virus variants. There could be a genetic component that influences the recognition receptors of the inflammatory cascade. The high affinity of the MHCII and TCR complex generated by the S protein could generate a higher production of inflammatory factors. The mutation of SOCS1 gene may decrease the ability to regulate the inflammatory cascade. The formation of a superantigen could amplify the inflammatory response. NK cells expands the immune response and could cause endothelial damage. The dysregulation of B lymphocytes produces autoantibodies that activate Fcγ receptors and also produce endothelial inflammation and complement activation, which contributes to increased hyperinflammation. Endothelia damaged perpetuates the inflammatory process. Endothelial dysfunction explain much of the signs and symptoms of the disease. TLR: Toll Like Receptor; MHC II: Major Histocompatibility Complex II; S protein: Spike protein; TCR: T cell receptors; MHC I: Major Histocompatibility Complex I; IL: interleukin; IFN: interferon; SOCS: suppression of cytokine signals.

Figure 2.
Theories that would explain the pathophysiology of MIS-C.

4. Clinical manifestation

4.1 Signs and symptoms

As described above, the onset of symptoms occurs weeks after exposure to the virus. During this period, the child is usually asymptomatic. When the disease manifests clinically, it starts with general symptoms that are not very specific. Fever is present and is one of the main criteria for diagnosing the syndrome. It is presented in all cases, being a requirement in all published clinical criteria. For CDC criteria fever >38°C must be at least 24 hrs., for WHO on the other hand it must be at least 3 days. Regardless of the criteria used, fever is a cardinal sign. The average duration is between 4 and 6 days. The early gastrointestinal symptoms are frequent to find, the series describe it in more than 60%. These include diffuse abdominal pain, vomiting, and diarrhea. Many of the children consult emergency services even with clinic suggestive of acute abdomen. Up to this point, the disease can mimic any common febrile gastrointestinal infection or can be similar to appendicitis. The involvement of skin is also frequent, and it is described between 45 and 75% of cases. It includes rash which is usually non-specific and generalized and swelling of the palms and hands with edema [14]. Another frequent clinical finding is the involvement of mucous membranes, which can vary between 30 and 75%, which includes inflammation of the labial mucosa presenting with edematous and reddened lips, and inflammation of lingual mucosa with a strawberry tongue, that resembles a Kawasaki Disease (KD)

[45, 46]. Ocular involvement can vary from 30 to 80% of cases, usually presenting as bilateral no purulent conjunctivitis. Other general symptoms may be present but in a low percentage. Neurocognitive involvement includes headache, lethargy, confusion, or irritability, which is described in less than 50% of cases [46]. Respiratory symptoms are rare during MIS-C, but may be present as a history of upper respiratory infection weeks prior to the onset of MIS-C symptoms. Lymphadenopathy is usually rare to find [47].

4.1.1 Severe presentation

So far, many children may express the disease with mild symptoms meeting the diagnostic criteria for CVC and WHO, but without cardiovascular compromise. The major problem is the group of patients who develops cardiovascular involvement. It is this involvement that reflects the severity of multisystemic inflammation and poses a potential life-threatening risk to affected pediatric population. These group of patient will need a pediatric critical care unit. It usually presents as shock, meeting most of the surviving sepsis campaign criteria, being difficult to differentiate it initially from a sepsis or a toxic shock since MIS-C usually is accompanied by cutaneous manifestations. Many children may show cardiovascular involvement due to cardiac dysfunction with or without coronary involvement. Coronary disease seems to be present more frequently than in KD. Arrhythmia is described but it is a less common presentation. Respiratory illness is rare in these critically ill patients and the need for invasive ventilatory support is often necessary for the management of pediatric shock and not for inflammation, damage or lung infection. The dysfunction of other organs is less frequent, but as it is generalized inflammatory multisystemic disease, there may be diffuse inflammation. This inflammation may present as serositis like pleurisy, pericardial effusion, and/or ascites. The liver can also be affected. There may be an increase in transaminases or even hepatitis. This condition is rare and fluctuates between 5 and 20% of cases. A neurologic clinic of mild symptoms was previously described at the beginning of symptoms; however when MIS-C is severe, it can severely compromise the central nervous system. The disease may present with encephalopathy, meningeal inflammation, and seizures [48].

4.1.2 Presentation phenotypes

The spectrum of the disease ranges from mild to severe as described above. MIS-C is new, so the factors that cause a child to evolve from mild-to-severe disease with cardiovascular involvement are still unknown. It is likely that laboratory tests that show a greater range of general inflammation are more frequently present in cases that are going to evolve to severe (3.2 laboratory tests); however, the severity of the disease is determined by cardiovascular involvement and presence of shock rather than by the results of laboratory tests [49]. What has been seen is that there are phenotypes resulting from associations combining the severity of the clinical presentation, the KD criteria, and the presence of shock. Then, we could classify the phenotype in three main forms: MIS-C phenotype KD without shock; MIS-C phenotype shock/myocarditis (with or without KD); and MIS-C phenotype without KD or shock.

MIS-C phenotype KD without shock. This is a group of children who, regardless of age, meet the WHO or CDC criteria for MIS-C, in which the clinical presentation fully or partially fulfills the diagnostic criteria for KD. These patients may have clinical and laboratory signs of general inflammation and even organ dysfunction or cardiac inflammation, but do not present with hypotension or signs of shock. Their laboratory tests show general and non-specific inflammation, but show no evidence of hypoperfusion.

MIS-C phenotype shock/myocarditis (with or without KD). These patients, who meet WHO and CDC criteria for MIS-C, show hypotension or evidence of shock regardless of the KD criteria. Then, we can have patients in shock with mucosal and cutaneous involvement like KD, but also patients in shock who do not show any Kawasaki signs. In them, the cardiovascular compromise can manifest as shock, by the criteria of the surviving sepsis campaign, or as myocarditis. Laboratory tests appear to show higher ranges of generic and cardiac inflammation. It is important to recognize this group of patients since they are children who require advanced monitoring and management of shock in an Intensive Care Unit (ICU).

MIS-C phenotype without KD or shock. These children also meet WHO and CDC criteria for MIS-C, but they have no clinical criteria for KD or clinical or laboratory evidence of hypoperfusion, shock or myocarditis. These patients, like the previous ones, present multisystem inflammation and organ systems involved, but without cardiovascular involvement.

All the groups have in common a generalized systemic inflammation, initiated as fever and gastrointestinal symptoms, defining their phenotypes in a few days. It is important to note that coronary alterations can be present in any of the groups. Coronary alterations are rare to observe in children, so it denotes severity of the disease, independent of filling the KD criteria and even without hypotension or shock. In summary, the clinical presentation of MIS-C can be very variable. Most children have a mild multisystemic inflammatory compromise without shock; however, the recognition of cardiovascular involvement is critical. Children with Shock (with or without KD criteria) are the group of patients that will require advanced critical care support, including advanced monitoring and in some cases connection to invasive mechanical ventilation. The pediatric population with an clinical presentation of shock are the children with the highest risk of morbidity and mortality.

4.2 Laboratory test

Laboratory tests reflect children's severe inflammatory involvement. Abnormal level of blood cell counts is one of the most frequent findings. The blood count shows elevation of white blood cells of neutrophilic predominance; however, the presence of lymphopenia is described as even more frequent, up to 80–95% of cases. Moderate anemia and thrombocytopenia can be observed in many cases and can be seen in 70 to 80%. The elevation of inflammatory parameters is relevant when making the diagnosis of MIS-C and is present in the diagnostic criteria of all clinical guidelines. There is an elevation of general inflammatory parameters and also of specific cardiac parameters. The rise of C-reactive protein (CRP) into bacterial range occurs up to 90–100%. Erythrocyte sedimentation rate (ESR) is another result that is elevated up to 80%. Procalcitonin also rises up in bacterial ranges [9, 47]. Elevation of other acute phase reactants such as ferritin, dimer D, and fibrinogen also occurs in 60 to 80% of MIS-C. Hypoalbuminemia is a common finding. As stated, when signs and symptoms were described, MIS-C can present with or without shock. Patients with shock have a greater elevation of inflammatory parameters compared to children without shock, so it could be assumed that these elevated parameters are related to the severity of the disease [50, 51]. Regarding interleukins, in MIS-C there is a severe elevation of Interleukin (IL) 6. It is interesting to note that although the elevation of IL6 is severe

Evidence of SARS-CoV-2 infection	Polymerase chain reaction (PCR)
	Serology (IGM/IGG)
	Antigen test
Inflammatory markers	C-reactive protein
	Erythrocyte sedimentation rate (ESR)
	Procalcitonin
	Ferritin
	Albumin
Hematology and coagulation	Hemogram
	D-dimer
	Fibrinogen
	Prothrombin time
	Partial thromboplastin time
Cardiac inflammation	Troponin T
	Creatine kinase
	Creatine kinase-MB
	B-type natriuretic peptide
Perfusion and organ dysfunction	Lactate
	Venous and arterial gases
	Creatinine and Ureic Nitrogen
	Transaminases
Other focus of infection	Blood cultures
	Urine and urine cultures
	Viral respiratory panel.
	Others according to symptoms
Images	Chest X-ray
	Echocardiography
	Others according to sign and symptoms

Table 1.
Tests required in MIS-C.

due to the large systemic inflammatory process that occurs in MIS-C, when compared to the IL6 measurements of pediatric septic shock, the latter are greater. This suggests that although the pathophysiological basis of MIS-C is immune-mediated, it is likely that IL6 is not the main interleukin mediating the disease [52]. Elevated cardiac inflammatory parameters seem to be important when making the diagnosis of pediatric inflammatory syndrome associated with COVID-19, since the heart is one of the main organs affected. Between 60 and 90% of patients with MIS-C can elevate troponins and/or pro BNP. As in general inflammatory parameters, cardiac laboratory elevation is greater in patients with shock than without it. The laboratory tests requested in children with MIS-C are shown in **Table 1**.

4.3 Images

There are no specific altered images in MIS-C. Chest X-ray shows no specific findings. Although infiltrates, consolidation or atelectasis may be observed, most of the patients have no acute respiratory clinic, so the most frequent finding is a normal chest X-ray. If X-ray shows pulmonary alteration, it may be a consequence of the SARS-CoV2 infection that occurred prior to MIS-C. It is rare to see a patient with an altered chest X-ray who is simultaneously in a multisystem inflammatory process, since MIS-C occurs weeks after the respiratory infection as explained above. It is possible to find pleural effusion as part of the inflammatory disease. One of the initial symptoms of the disease is abdominal pain that can even mimic an acute abdomen, so abdominal ultrasound is a study frequently requested. Like chest X-ray, abdominal images are non-specific for the disease, showing alterations that are mainly a consequence of a diffuse inflammatory process. It can observe ascites, free fluid, ileitis, and mesenteric adenopathy/adenitis. Chest or abdomen computed tomography (CT) does not show specific alterations. The most altered image study is echocardiography. There is no specific finding in cardiac ultrasound, being able to find multiple alterations alone or associated. Left ventricle (LV) dysfunction can be found up to 40% of patients with MIS-C. If the disease presents clinically as shock, depression of LV function is more frequent, being present in up to 60% of these severe cases. Heart valve diseases such as mitral or tricuspid regurgitation also may be found. Pericardial effusion can be seen, and as well as pleural effusion and ascites, it is due to a generalized inflammatory process with serositis. One of the most important findings of the disease is the alteration of the coronary arteries (CA). This type of alteration is very rare in children, with KD being one of the few pediatric diseases in which it is present. CA abnormalities include dilation or aneurysm. This alteration may be present up to 25% of mild cases and even up to 50% in severe cases with shock. CA assessment is based on Z-scores used in KD [53–55]. Performing cardiac nuclear magnetic resonance imaging (MRI) is rare, but when it has been done, myocardial edema and abnormal strain is described, compatible with a generalized cardiac inflammatory process [56].

5. Diagnosis

5.1 Case definition

The CDC or WHO criteria are the most commonly used case definition. Regardless of the institution that defines the case, all definitions have some pillars to make the diagnosis. The first is a pediatric patient with fever. The second is to have inflammation of at least two systems, by clinical presentation or by laboratory test. The third is to have altered laboratory parameters that show a systemic and generalized process of inflammation. The fourth is to have ruled out any infection that is not COVID and finally any epidemiological association with SARS-CoV2 infection [7, 8]. Case definition criteria are shown in **Tables 2** and **3**.

The criteria can be modified over time as there is more knowledge of the syndrome. CDC will change the current case definition in 2023. Among main changes are fever lasting >24 hrs. Will be changed by subjective or documented fever >38.0°C. Illness requiring hospitalization will be changed for severe illness that requires hospitalization

1	Age 0 to 19 years
2	Fever for ≥3 days
3	Clinical signs of multisystem involvement (at least 2 of the following):
	Rash, bilateral no purulent conjunctivitis, or mucocutaneous inflammation signs (oral, hands, or feet)
	• Hypotension or shock
	• Cardiac dysfunction, pericarditis, valvulitis, or coronary abnormalities
	(including echocardiographic findings or elevated troponin/BNP)
	• Evidence of coagulopathy (prolonged PT or PTT; elevated D-dimer)
	• Acute gastrointestinal symptoms (diarrhea, vomiting, or abdominal pain)
4	Elevated markers of inflammation (e.g., ESR, CRP, or procalcitonin)
5	No other obvious microbial cause of inflammation.
	(including bacterial sepsis and staphylococcal/streptococcal toxic shock syndromes)
6	Evidence of SARS-CoV-2 infection (any of the following):
	• Positive SARS-CoV-2 RT-PCR
	• Positive serology
	• Positive antigen test
	• Contact with an individual with COVID-19

World Health Organization [7].
BNP: B-type natriuretic peptide. PT: Prothrombin time. PTT: Partial thromboplastin time. ESR: Erythrocyte sedimentation rate. CRP: c-reactive protein. PCR: Polymerase chain reaction.

Table 2.
WHO MIS-C case definition (all criteria are required).

1	Fever >38.0°C or subjective fever lasting >24 hrs.
2	Illness requiring hospitalization
3	Laboratory evidence of inflammation (e.g., CRP, ESR)
4	Multisystem organ involvement (at least 2 of the following):
	• Cardiac (e.g., shock, Troponin elevation, BNP elevation, abnormal echo, arrhythmia)
	• Dermatologic (e.g., rash, mucocutaneous lesions)
	• Gastrointestinal (e.g., diarrhea, bilirubin or liver enzyme elevation)
	• Hematologic (e.g., D-dimer elevation, thrombophilia, thrombocytopenia)
	• Neurologic, Renal, Respiratory.
3	Positive for current or recent SARS-CoV-2 infection by PCR, serology, or antigen test; or exposure to a suspected or confirmed COVID-19 case within the 4 weeks prior to the onset symptoms.

Health Alert Network (HAN) [8].
CRP: c-reactive protein, ESR: erythrocyte sedimentation rate, BNP: B-type natriuretic peptide, and PCR: polymerase chain reaction.

Table 3.
2020 CDC MIS-C case definition (all criteria are required).

and may result in death. Laboratory makers of inflammation will be limited to just CRP >3 mg/dl. Shock will appear as a separate criterion of cardiac involvement. Coronary involvement will include coronary dilatation/aneurysm and left ventricular ejection <55%. Dermatological criteria will be more explicit: oral mucosal inflammation, conjunctivitis/conjunctival injection, or extremity findings (erythema, edema). Gastrointestinal criteria will be limited to abdominal pain, vomiting, or diarrhea. Renal, respiratory, and neurologic organ system involvement will be removed.

5.2 Differential diagnosis

Because it is a disease that can have many clinical presentations, there are many possible differential diagnoses but there are some of them that are essential to rule out. In many cases, the disease simulates sepsis or septic shock, both by its clinical presentation or by laboratory tests in ranges that simulate bacterial infection. The main difference is that in MIS-C there is no bacterial infectious focus and that no infectious agent is isolated. The association with SARS-CoV-2 as the only infectious agent it is absolutely necessary.

5.2.1 Infectious inflammatory diseases

Appendicitis: MIS-C may present as acute abdomen. Fever added to abdominal pain and tests in bacterial range make appendicitis difficult to rule it out. At the beginning of the pandemic, cases of children undergoing laparoscopies for suspected appendicitis were reported in which normal appendices were found. To dismiss the diagnosis of appendicitis, an abdominal image (ultrasound or CT) is required. In MIS-C, this image shows non-specific abdominal inflammatory findings but no inflammation of the cecal appendage.

Sepsis y Septic Shock: It is one of the main diagnoses to discard. Aforesaid, MIS-C simulates a bacterial infection, with fever and laboratory parameters in bacterial range, even in severe cases of MIS-C may show evidence of shock. That is why many established protocols suggest the initiation of antibiotics empirically and then suspend them once an infectious focus has been ruled out. Unlike septic shock, MIS-C does not have a specific infectious focus and bacterial infectious agents cannot be identified. It is necessary to take cultures to rule out the main bacterial pediatric infectious diseases. At least blood cultures are required to rule out bacteremia and complete urine with urine culture to rule out urinary focus. Other studies may be added depending on the clinical presentation. Intestinal pathogens can be searched if gastrointestinal clinic predominates. Study of cerebrospinal fluid can be studied if the predominant clinic is neurological. Other studies depend on each case. With negative cultures and once any clinical focus is dismissed, the bacterial cause of the inflammatory process should be ruled out.

Toxic Shock Syndrome (TSS): It has many similarities with MIS-C, since they share the multisystem inflammation, laboratory tests in similarly high ranges and the skin involvement. The main difference between both conditions is the presence of a clinical focus and the bacterial origin of the (TSS). Cultures are required to determine staphylococcal or streptococcal infection.

Other viral infections: There are viral pathogens that can cause systemic inflammation and skin involvement, including this adenovirus, cytomegalovirus, Epstein Barr virus, enterovirus, and parvovirus among others. Infection with these agents often occurs in immunosuppressed patients. In general, these viral infections do not produce an elevation of inflammatory parameters in bacterial range. If the suspicion exists, molecular study by polymerase chain reaction is necessary to confirm the presence of this viral infection.

5.2.2 Immune-mediated inflammatory diseases

Kawasaki disease: This is a challenge as they share a large number of clinical and laboratory elements. The situation becomes more difficult if the MIS-C does not meet all the KD criteria, with the incomplete Kawasaki being more difficult to distinguish from a MIS-C. The keys to differentiate them could be the gastrointestinal symptoms that are more frequent in MIS-C, cardiovascular dysfunction, and shock that are rare in KD (KD shock syndrome has an incidence rate of only 3.3–7% of KD cases) [57], high inflammatory parameters in laboratory tests associated with lymphopenia most common in MIS-C and the temporal association or evidence of exposure to SARS-CoV-2 [25].

Systemic lupus erythematosus (SLE): Like MIS-C, SLE is a multisystem immune process which can have skin involvement and that occurs with elevation of inflammatory parameters often in bacterial ranges. One of the elements to be taken into consideration to differentiate these diseases is age, being SLE more frequent in adolescent patients; female sex that is predominant in SLE, renal involvement that is much less frequent in MIS-C; and the neurological compromise that is most associated with SLE.

Hemophagocytic lymphohistiocytosis (HLH): Macrophage activation syndrome (MAS).

This disease shares characteristics with MIS-C, both in multiorgan involvement and in laboratory parameters. It usually occurs in patients with a history of immune-rheumatologic diseases, but can also be triggered by viral or bacterial infectious diseases in previously healthy patients. There are diagnostic criteria published by the histiocyte society. Fever, high C-reactive protein, high ferritin, and thrombocytopenia are elements that it shares with MIS-C; however, the compromise of other lines of the blood count as well as the increase in triglycerides is not common in MIS-C. One of the most important tests for HLH/MAS is the elevation of soluble CD25, which does not occur in MIS-C.

6. Treatment

Treatment has two goals. The first is to stop hyperinflammation and the second is to treat cardiovascular complications that could be associated in severe cases. At the time of this publication, there are no randomized controlled studies evaluating the treatment of MIS-C.

6.1 Treatment of hyperinflammation

Many ways to immunomodulate the disease are described, most of them initially borrowed from Kawasaki disease and other hyperinflammatory syndromes. They could be grouped into three approaches: the use of intravenous immunoglobulin (IVIG), the use of steroids, and the use of biological drugs.

6.1.1 IVIG and steroids

VIG is the most commonly used drug to modulate MIS-C followed by glucocorticoids. There are few comparative studies between the use of IVIG and steroids, and their results are contradictory. On the one hand, some studies would suggest that the joint use of both therapies appears to have some impact on signs or symptoms, as well as in severe cardiovascular evolution (v/s IVIG alone). On the other hand, some publications suggest that patients who meet the WHO criteria for MIS-C are treated with glucocorticoids and they would have a possible benefit (v/s IVIG alone). Moreover, other studies show no difference between using IVIG alone, steroids alone, or the two therapies together. In view of the lack of evidence, but with the clarity that patients respond to immunomodulatory therapy, scientific societies have published treatment recommendations. American College of Rheumatology (ACR) recommends the use of IVIG as a first line in all patients with MIS-C with addition of glucocorticoids in the presence of shock, organ-threatening disease or refractory disease. There are countless protocols, adapted according to each local reality. The recommended doses of IVIG are 2gr/kg/day once. Methylprednisolone doses vary according to protocols between 2 and 10 mg/k/day for 3 days. In general, patients respond to the use of IVIG and steroids. Patients who maintain fever and elevated inflammatory parameters are considered refractory. In this type of patients, the use of biological drugs is considered [58].

6.1.2 Biological drugs

The use of biological therapy as rescue in patients refractory to IVIG/steroid treatment is described in many protocols. Like other therapies, these drugs were extrapolated from the treatment of KD and other diseases with systemic inflammatory processes. In order to block the effect of IL-1B, anakinra (an IL-1 receptor blocker) has been used. Another IL receptor blockade described is IL-6 by tocilizumab. Infliximab is another monoclonal antibody, used in refractory KD, to stop the effect of tumor necrosis factor alpha (TNFa) [59]. This drug is also described as a therapeutic tool in refractory MIS-C. As shown in **Figure 2**, the pathophysiology of MIS-C is complex,. Trying to stop an inflammatory cascade by blocking a single pathway seems unlikely. IL6 is elevated in both MIS-C and pediatric septic patients (both diseases with immune dysregulation). Septic patients have higher IL-6 plasmatic levels and have good outcomes without using interleukin blockade, suggesting that there is no clear role of some IL6 in the pathophysiology of MIS-C [52]. The use of biological drugs is continuously studied for this pathology.

6.2 Treatment of cardiovascular complications

Severe MIS-C can lead to severe cardiovascular dysfunction that can be life threatening for children. Endothelial involvement and cardiac dysfunction (with or without coronary alteration) can lead to hypotension, hypoperfusion, and dysfunction of other organs. It must be managed as shock, and in many cases it requires volume, vasoactive drugs, and even connection to mechanical ventilation as part of shock management. Due to the compromise of vascular tone, norepinephrine is indicated. If there is cardiac dysfunction, epinephrine should be associated. In the case of coronary alterations, anti-inflammatory and antiplatelet treatment with acetylsalicylic acid is used in MIS-C protocols. This management was extrapolated from KD protocols. Although abnormal coagulation parameters are frequently reported, thrombotic or embolic events were rare, in contrast to adult COVID-19 [59, 60]. Other management of vascular complications includes the possibility of thrombosis. High D-dimer is frequently found in this disease and could be associated with greater hypercoagulability, which is why many protocols include the use of anticoagulation such as enoxaparin until the inflammatory process and D-dimer go down.

7. Prognosis

MIS-C can be potentially life threatening. The need for admission to ICU was described, 40% of patients needs inotropic drugs, 15% is connected to mechanical ventilation, and even needs for extracorporeal oxygenation membrane (ECMO) have been reported. Despite what has been described, MIS-C is a disease with low mortality, less than 2%. Recovery from acute organ dysfunctions occurs quickly with a median ICU length of stay of 5 days. Recovery from sequelae is close to 6 months; however, there are reports of poor exercise tolerance. The disease was found less than 3 years ago, so large follow-up studies of these patients are needed to determine the long-term outcomes of these children [61].

8. Prevention

Early recognition of the disease is fundamental through the signs and symptoms described, in order to perform a precocious immunomodulatory treatment that allows the control of the disease and better outcomes. Clinical alert should be maintained as long as SARS-CoV-2 is circulating within the population. While clinics maintain the search for MIS-C in febrile children, it is necessary at the same time preventing waves of new viral variants and the emergence of high rates of MIS-C which until now remains low. It seems that the only way to prevent the disease is to maintain vaccination of the entire population. SARS-CoV-2 is a virus that is here to stay, but can be controlled by vaccination. The massive inoculation of the population led the virus to mutate into variants that are apparently less susceptible to producing severe inflammatory phenomena in children, as seen in the omicron wave. If the world population lowers its vaccination rates, it is likely that the virus will continue to mutate, giving the possibility of new variants that could have the potential to cause higher MIS-C rates again. It is possible that areas with less economic development and therefore less access to vaccines keep low vaccination rates. In those places, the possibility of the appearance of new variants could be high. Efforts should also be maintained for the implementation of the vaccine at all pediatric ages, given the actual change in the epidemiology of MIS-C at younger ages without access to vaccination.

9. Conclusion

MIS-C is a newly emerging disease that shares its clinical presentation simulating other serious pediatric diseases, which implies a diagnostic challenge for clinicians. Its pathophysiology is not well known but it is clear that it is a post-infectious immune syndrome. Life threatening is given by cardiac and vascular involvement. In the post-COVID era, the effort must then focus on maintaining the clinical search for the disease, maintaining vaccination of both adults and children, and in prioritizing less developed countries with poor access to vaccination.

Author details

Felipe Yagnam Rojas[1,2,3]

1 Pediatric Intensive Care Unit, Dr. Exequiel Gonzalez Cortés Children's Hospital, Santiago, Chile

2 Pediatric Intensive Care Unit, Clínica Universidad de Los Andes, Santiago, Chile

3 Department of Pediatrics, Faculty of Medicine, University of Chile, Santiago, Chile

*Address all correspondence to: felipeyagnam@gmail.com

IntechOpen

© 2023 The Author(s). Licensee IntechOpen. This chapter is distributed under the terms of the Creative Commons Attribution License (http://creativecommons.org/licenses/by/3.0), which permits unrestricted use, distribution, and reproduction in any medium, provided the original work is properly cited.

References

[1] World Health Organization. Director-General's remarks at the media briefing on 2019-nCoV on 11 February 2020. Available from: http://www.who.int/dg/speeches/detail/who-director-general-s-remarks-at-the-media-briefing-on-2019-ncov-on-11-february-2020 [Accessed on Dec 18, 2020]

[2] Shahid Z, Kalayanamitra R, McClafferty B, et al. COVID-19 and older adults: What we know. Journal of the American Geriatrics Society. 2020;**68**(5):926-929. DOI: 10.1111/jgs.16472

[3] Dionne A, Son MBF, Randolph AG. An update on multisystem inflammatory syndrome in children related to SARS-CoV-2. The Pediatric Infectious Disease Journal. 2022;**41**(1):e6-e9. DOI: 10.1097/INF.0000000000003393

[4] King MA, Matos RI, Hamele MT, et al. PICU in the MICU: How adult ICUs can support Pediatric Care in Public Health Emergencies. Chest. 2022;**161**(5):1297-1305. DOI: 10.1016/j.chest.2021.12.648

[5] Viner RM, Whittaker E. Kawasaki-like disease: Emerging complication during the COVID-19 pandemic. Lancet. 2020;**395**(10239):1741-1743. DOI: 10.1016/S0140-6736(20)31129-6

[6] Verdoni L, Mazza A, Gervasoni A, at al. An outbreak of severe Kawasaki-like disease at the Italian epicentre of the SARS-CoV-2 epidemic: An observational cohort study. Lancet. 2020;**395**(10239):1771-1778. DOI: 10.1016/S0140-6736(20)31103-X

[7] World Health Organization. Novel Coronavirus (2019-nCoV) technical guidance. Available from: https://www.who.int/emergencies/diseases/novel-coronavirus-2019/technical-guidance [Accessed: December 18, 2022]

[8] Health Alert Network (HAN): Multisystem Inflammatory Syndrome in Children (MIS-C) Associated with Coronavirus Disease 2019 (COVID-19). Available from: https://emergency.cdc.gov/han/2020/han00432.asp [Accessed: December 18, 2022]

[9] Son MB, Friedman K. COVID-19: Multisystem inflammatory syndrome in children (MIS-C) clinical features, evaluation, and diagnosis. In: Post TW, editor. UpToDate. Waltham, MA: UpToDate Inc.; 2022. Available from: https://www.uptodate.com [Accessed: January 02, 2023]

[10] Chang JC, Son MBF. When vaccine adverse event reporting generates hope, not fear. Lancet Child and Adolescent Health. 2022;**6**(5):281-282. DOI: 10.1016/S2352-4642(22)00061-X

[11] Dufort EM, Koumans EH, Chow EJ, et al. Multisystem Inlamatory syndrome in children in New York state. The New England Journal of Medicine. 2020;**383**:347

[12] Miller AD, Zambrano LD, Yousaf AR, et al. Multisystem inflammatory syndrome in children in united state. Clinical Infectious Diseases. 2022;**75**:e1165

[13] Payne AB, Gilani Z, Gosfred-Cato S, et al. Incidence of multisystem inflammatory syndrome in children among US persons infected with SARS-CoV-2. JAMA Network Open. 2021;**4**:e2116420

[14] Feldstein LR, Rose EB, Horwitz SM, et al. Multisystem inflammatory syndrome in US children and

adolescents. The New England Journal of Medicine. 2020;**383**:334

[15] Davies P, Evans C, Kanthimathinathan HK, et al. Intensive care admissions of children with pediatric inflammatory multisystem syndrome temporally associated with SARS-CoV-2 (PIMS-TS) in the UK.: A multicenter observational study. Lancet Child and Adolescent Health. 2020;**4**:699

[16] Stierman B, Abrams JY, Godfred-Cato SE, et al. Racial and ethnic disparities in multisystem inflammatory syndrome in children in the United States, march 2020 to February 2021. The Pediatric Infectious Disease Journal. 2021;**40**(11):e400-e406

[17] Coffin SE, Rubin D. Yes, children can transmit COVID, but we need not fear. JAMA Pediatrics. 2021;**175**(11):1110-1112. DOI: 10.1001/jamapediatrics.2021.2767

[18] Lopez L, Burgner D, Glover C, et al. Lower risk of multi-system inflammatory syndrome in children (MIS-C) with the omicron variant. Lancet Regional Health–Western Pacific. 2022;**27**:100604. DOI: 10.1016/j.lanwpc.2022.100604

[19] Cohen JM, Carter MJ, Cheung CR, et al. Lower risk of multisystem inflammatory syndrome in children (MIS-C) with the delta and omicron variants of SARS-CoV-2. Clinical Infectious Diseases. 8 Feb 2023;**76**(3):e518-e521. DOI: 10.1093/cid/ciac553

[20] Levy N, Koppel JH, Kaplan O, et al. Severity and incidence of multisystem inflammatory syndrome in children during 3 SARS-CoV-2 pandemic waves in Israel. Journal of the American Medical Association. 2022;**327**(24):2452-2454. DOI: 10.1001/jama.2022.8025

[21] Holm M, Espenhain L, Glenthoj J, et al. Risk and phenotype of multisystem inflammatory syndrome in vaccinated and unvaccinated Danish children before and during the omicron wave. JAMA Pediatrics. 2022;176(8):821-823. DOI: 10.1001/jamapediatrics.2022.2206. Erratum in: JAMA Pediatr. 2022;176(8):829

[22] David J, Hradsky O, Jabandziev P, et al. Impact of SARS-CoV-2 variants on the incidence of paediatric inflammatory multisystem syndrome (PIMS-TS). Journal of Paediatrics and Child Health. 2022;**58**(10):1901-1903. DOI: 10.1111/jpc.16204

[23] Shingleton J, Williams H, Oligbu G, et al. The changing epidemiology of PIMS-TS across COVID-19 waves: Prospective national surveillance, January 2021 to July 2022, England. Journal of Infections. 2022;**85**(6):702-769. DOI: 10.1016/j.jinf.2022.10.017

[24] Whittaker R, Greve-Isdahl M, Bøås H, et al. COVID-19 hospitalization among children <18 years by variant wave in Norway. Pediatrics. 2022;**150**(3):e2022057564. DOI: 10.1542/peds.2022-057564

[25] Sharma C, Ganigara M, Galeotti C, et al. Multisystem inflammatory syndrome in children and Kawasaki disease: A critical comparison. Nature Reviews Rheumatology. 2021;**17**:731-748. DOI: 10.1038/s41584-021-00709-9

[26] Bartsch YC, Wang C, Zohar T, Fischinger S, et al. Humoral signatures of protective and pathological SARS-CoV-2 infection in children. Nature Medicine. 2021;**27**(3):454-462. DOI: 10.1038/s41591-021-01263-3

[27] Yonker LM, Gilboa T, Ogata AF, et al. Multisystem inflammatory syndrome

in children is driven by zonulin-dependent loss of gut mucosal barrier. The Journal of Clinical Investigation. 2021;**131**(14):e149633. DOI: 10.1172/JCI149633

[28] Ramaswamy A, Brodsky NN, Sumida TS, et al. Immune dysregulation and autoreactivity correlate with disease severity in SARS-CoV-2-associated multisystem inflammatory syndrome in children. Immunity. 2021;**54**(5):1083-1095.e7. DOI: 10.1016/j.immuni.2021.04.003

[29] Perez-Toledo M, Faustini SE, Jossi SE, et al. SARS-CoV-2-specific IgG1/IgG3 but not IgM in children with Pediatric inflammatory multi-system syndrome. Pediatric Allergy and Immunology. 2021;**32**(5):1125-1129. DOI: 10.1111/pai.13504

[30] Gruber CN, Patel RS, Trachtman R, et al. Mapping systemic inflammation and antibody responses in multisystem inflammatory syndrome in children (MIS-C). Cell. 2020;**183**(4):982-995.e14. DOI: 10.1016/j.cell.2020.09.034

[31] Rostad CA, Chahroudi A, Mantus G, et al. Quantitative SARS-CoV-2 serology in children with multisystem inflammatory syndrome (MIS-C). Pediatrics. 2020;**146**(6):e2020018242. DOI: 10.1542/peds.2020-018242

[32] Weisberg SP, Connors TJ, Zhu Y, et al. Distinct antibody responses to SARS-CoV-2 in children and adults across the COVID-19 clinical spectrum. Nature Immunology. 2021;**22**(1):25-31. DOI: 10.1038/s41590-020-00826-9

[33] Mateus J, Grifoni A, Tarke A, et al. Selective and cross-reactive SARS-CoV-2 T cell epitopes in unexposed humans. Science. 2020;**370**(6512):89-94. DOI: 10.1126/science.abd3871

[34] Grifoni A, Weiskopf D, Ramirez SI, et al. Targets of T cell responses to SARS-CoV-2 coronavirus in humans with COVID-19 disease and unexposed individuals. Cell. 2020;**181**(7):1489-1501.e15. DOI: 10.1016/j.cell.2020.05.015

[35] Sermet-Gaudelus I, Temmam S, Huon C, et al. Prior infection by seasonal coronaviruses, as assessed by serology, does not prevent SARS-CoV-2 infection and disease in children, France, April to June 2020. Euro Surveillance. 2021;**26**(13):2001782. DOI: 10.2807/1560-7917.ES.2021.26.13.2001782

[36] Vella LA, Giles JR, Baxter AE, et al. Deep immune profiling of MIS-C demonstrates marked but transient immune activation compared to adult and pediatric COVID-19. Science Immunology. 2021;**6**(57):eabf7570. DOI: 10.1126/sciimmunol.abf7570

[37] Vojdani A, Vojdani E, Kharrazian D. Reaction of human monoclonal antibodies to SARS-CoV-2 proteins with tissue antigens: Implications for autoimmune diseases. Frontiers in Immunology. 2021;**11**:617089. DOI: 10.3389/fimmu.2020.617089

[38] Whitworth H, Sartain SE, Kumar R, et al. Rate of thrombosis in children and adolescents hospitalized with COVID-19 or MIS-C. Blood. 2021;**138**(2):190-198. DOI: 10.1182/blood.2020010218

[39] Noval Rivas M, Porritt RA, Cheng MH, et al. COVID-19-associated multisystem inflammatory syndrome in children (MIS-C): A novel disease that mimics toxic shock syndrome-the superantigen hypothesis. The Journal of Allergy and Clinical Immunology. 2021;**147**(1):57-59. DOI: 10.1016/j.jaci.2020.10.008

[40] Porritt RA, Paschold L, Rivas MN, et al. HLA class I-associated expansion

of TRBV11-2 T cells in multisystem inflammatory syndrome in children. The Journal of Clinical Investigation. 2021;**131**(10):e146614. DOI: 10.1172/JCI146614

[41] Cheng MH, Zhang S, Porritt RA, et al. Superantigenic character of an insert unique to SARS-CoV-2 spike supported by skewed TCR repertoire in patients with hyperinflammation. Proceedings of the National Academy of Sciences of the United States of America. 2020;**117**(41):25254-25262. DOI: 10.1073/pnas.2010722117

[42] Chou J, Platt CD, Habiballah S, et al. Mechanisms underlying genetic susceptibility to multisystem inflammatory syndrome in children (MIS-C). The Journal of Allergy and Clinical Immunology. 2021;**148**(3):732-738.e1. DOI: 10.1016/j.jaci.2021.06.024

[43] Lee PY, Day-Lewis M, Henderson LA, et al. Distinct clinical and immunological features of SARS-CoV-2-induced multisystem inflammatory syndrome in children. The Journal of Clinical Investigation. 2020;**130**(11):5942-5950. DOI: 10.1172/JCI141113

[44] Peart Akindele N, Kouo T, Karaba AH, et al. Distinct cytokine and chemokine dysregulation in hospitalized children with acute coronavirus disease 2019 and multisystem inflammatory syndrome with similar levels of nasopharyngeal severe acute respiratory syndrome coronavirus 2 shedding. The Journal of Infectious Diseases. 2021;**224**(4):606-615. DOI: 10.1093/infdis/jiab285

[45] Yagnam RF, Izquierdo CG, Villena MR, González MC, Drago-T M. Pediatric multisystemic inflammatory syndrome temporarily associated with COVID-19: Clinical characteristics and management in a pediatric critical care unit. Andes Pediatrica: Revista Chilena de Pediatria. 2021;**92**(3):395-405. English, Spanish. DOI: 10.32641/andespediatr.v92i3.3333

[46] LaRovere KL, Riggs BJ, Poussaint TY, et al. Neurologic involvement in children and adolescents hospitalized in the United States for COVID-19 or multisystem inflammatory syndrome. JAMA Neurology. 2021;**78**(5):536-547. DOI: 10.1001/jamaneurol.2021.0504

[47] Whittaker E, Bamford A, Kenny J, et al. Clinical characteristics of 58 children with a Pediatric inflammatory multisystem syndrome temporally associated with SARS-CoV-2. Journal of the American Medical Association. 2020;**324**(3):259-269. DOI: 10.1001/jama.2020.10369

[48] Hoste L, Van Paemel R, Haerynck F. Multisystem inflammatory syndrome in children related to COVID-19: A systematic review. European Journal of Pediatrics. 2021;**180**(7):2019-2034. DOI: 10.1007/s00431-021-03993-5

[49] Rao S, Jing N, Liu X, et al. Clinical Subphenotypes of Multisystem Inflammatory Syndrome in Children: An EHR-based cohort study from the RECOVER program. medRxiv [Preprint]. 2022:2022.09.26.22280364. DOI: 10.1101/2022.09.26.22280364

[50] Rey-Jurado E, Espinosa Y, Astudillo C, et al. Deep immunophenotyping reveals biomarkers of multisystemic inflammatory syndrome in children in a Latin American cohort. The Journal of Allergy and Clinical Immunology. 2022;**150**(5):1074-1085.e11. DOI: 10.1016/j.jaci.2022.09.006

[51] Abrams JY, Oster ME, Godfred-Cato SE, et al. Factors linked to severe outcomes in multisystem

inflammatory syndrome in children (MIS-C) in the USA: A retrospective surveillance study. Lancet Child and Adolescent Health. 2021;**5**(5):323-331. DOI: 10.1016/S2352-4642(21)00050-X

[52] Diaz F, Bustos BR, Yagnam F, et al. Comparison of Interleukin-6 plasma concentration in multisystem inflammatory syndrome in children associated with SARS-CoV-2 and Pediatric sepsis. Frontiers in Pediatrics. 2021;**9**:756083. DOI: 10.3389/fped.2021.756083

[53] Belhadjer Z, Méot M, Bajolle F, et al. Acute heart failure in multisystem inflammatory syndrome in children in the context of global SARS-CoV-2 pandemic. Circulation. 2020;**142**(5):429-436. DOI: 10.1161/CIRCULATIONAHA.120.048360

[54] Matsubara D, Kauffman HL, Wang Y, et al. Echocardiographic findings in Pediatric multisystem inflammatory syndrome associated with COVID-19 in the United States. Journal of the American College of Cardiology. 2020;**76**(17):1947-1961. DOI: 10.1016/j.jacc.2020.08.056

[55] Theocharis P, Wong J, Pushparajah K, et al. Multimodality cardiac evaluation in children and young adults with multisystem inflammation associated with COVID-19. European Heart Journal Cardiovascular Imaging. 2021;**22**(8):896-903. DOI: 10.1093/ehjci/jeaa212

[56] Blumfield E, Levin TL, Kurian J, et al. Imaging findings in multisystem inflammatory syndrome in children (MIS-C) associated with coronavirus disease (COVID-19). AJR. American Journal of Roentgenology. 2021;**216**(2):507-517. DOI: 10.2214/AJR.20.24032

[57] Kanegaye JT, Wilder MS, Molkara D, et al. Recognition of a Kawasaki disease shock syndrome. Pediatrics. 2009;**123**(5):e783-e789. DOI: 10.1542/peds.2008-1871

[58] Henderson LA, Canna SW, Friedman KG, et al. American College of Rheumatology Clinical Guidance for multisystem inflammatory syndrome in children associated with SARS-CoV-2 and Hyperinflammation in Pediatric COVID-19: Version 2. Arthritis & Rhematology. 2021;**73**(4):e13-e29. DOI: 10.1002/art.41616

[59] Mahmoud S, El-Kalliny M, Kotby A, El-Ganzoury M, Fouda E, Ibrahim H. Treatment of MIS-C in children and adolescents. Current Pediatrics Reports. 2022;**10**(1):1-10. DOI: 10.1007/s40124-021-00259-4

[60] Fontelo P, Bastola MM, Zheng Z, Baik SH. A review of thromboembolic events in hospitalized COVID-19 patients. Thrombosis Journal. 2021;**19**(1):47. DOI: 10.1186/s12959-021-00298-3

[61] Penner J, Abdel-Mannan O, Grant K, et al. 6-month multidisciplinary follow-up and outcomes of patients with paediatric inflammatory multisystem syndrome (PIMS-TS) at a UK tertiary paediatric hospital: A retrospective cohort study. Lancet Child and Adolescent Health. 2021;**5**(7):473-482. DOI: 10.1016/S2352-4642(21)00138-3

Section 3

Sequelaes from COVID-19

Chapter 3

Post-COVID Stroke and Rehabilitation: A Rising Concern

Thajus Asirvatham, Premraj Isaac Chandran and Ajay Boppana

Abstract

The study of the consequences following COVID infection to comprehend the long-term and after-effects of this lethal epidemic is an emerging area of interest. In the light of COVID's many known and unknow manifestations, life after COVID seems to be so unpredictable. To the best of their ability, biopsychosocial models have described the scope of the epidemic. Acute ischemic stroke (AIS) is one of the biggest consequences following COVID, albeit the underlying mechanisms are yet unknown. Research on the connection between COVID-19 infection and stroke is ongoing. We can obtain a better knowledge of the efficacy of rehabilitation by looking at the functional improvement of such a susceptible population following active rehabilitation services and by comprehending the likely predictors. To deliver the right care, these variables influencing functional gain must be quickly addressed. The goal of rehabilitation, an evidence-based, problem-solving approach, is to promote positive outcomes and demonstrate success. This chapter offers a perspective on the problems following a COVID stroke as well as the consequences of rehabilitation and its efficacy in promoting optimal functioning and raising general quality of life.

Keywords: COVID-19, stroke, rehabilitation, Qatar, function

1. Introduction

On January 30, 2020, the World Health Organization (WHO) deemed the COVID-19 outbreak a public health emergency of global significance. Since then, there has been a sharp increase in the pandemic's transmission and spread. Different strategies have been used to halt the infection's spread. Those impacted by the post-COVID-19 infection have had long-lasting effects of varying intensities. The post-pandemic severity levels appear to have had a negative impact on people's general quality of life. The incidence of stroke is currently one of the most common post-COVID consequences observed and studied. Stroke is a crippling ailment that ranks as the second greatest cause of mortality and a significant contributor to disability globally. Along with premorbid health traits and lifestyle, its incidence rises with age. The rise of cerebrovascular events (CVE) linked to COVID-19 is a new finding. Following COVID-19 infection, acute ischemic stroke (AIS) is now a serious consequence. In order to treat such diseases, rehabilitation is essential.

IntechOpen

Recovery from an infection or trauma requires a multi-disciplinary team approach known as rehabilitation. The main essential concepts of rehabilitation are to enable maximal function, enable return to employment, enable safe departure from the hospital to home, and facilitate reintegration into the community. In order to achieve the best results, rehabilitation goals in such a vulnerable population must be carefully evaluated and tailored. The necessity and demand for the right intervention are highest due to the rise in post-COVID stroke cases. This enables the fields of study and rehabilitation to examine the requirements and effects brought on by the illness. The consequences and repercussions of the illness have been the subject of numerous researches recently. However, the need for rehabilitation is brought on by the various clinical presentations. Investigating how the rehabilitation process might assist and permit enough functioning in such a vulnerable population becomes extremely important as a result.

2. Impact of COVID-19

The COVID-19 infection has already created enough havoc and commotion around the globe. Depending on the infection's severity and the amount of its dissemination, the effect may differ. To treat the weak and limit the spread of disease, however, the entire world returned with a range of strategies. Isolation, quarantine, and lockdowns have impacted the lives of millions of people, which has had a negative impact on the economy and general well-being [1, 2]. Critically ill patients and COVID-19 survivors are more likely to have preexisting disorders that make them disabled, including functional, social, and mental or psychological side effects from severe illness. This includes a typically gradual recovery that lowers overall quality of life [3].

Cerebrovascular events (CVE) were one of the COVID-19 infection's many post-infection consequences that were of major importance [4]. A significant COVID-19 disease consequence is still acute ischemic stroke. Even if there are more reports of these situations, it is still unclear what the underlying mechanisms are [5]. The incidence of acute ischemic stroke (AIS) linked to severe COVID-19 is rising quickly. Currently, research is being done on the underlying pathophysiological pathways linked to peripheral and central inflammation that cause ischemic strokes linked to COVID-19. The angiotensin-converting enzyme 2 (ACE2) receptors on epithelial and endothelial cells are known to bind to SARS-CoV2, and this binding results in hypercoagulability, clot formation, and ultimately AIS [6]. Systemic immunity-mediated hyperinflammation, endothelitis, deregulation of the renin-angiotensin-aldosterone system (RAAS) in the central nervous system, oxidative stress, and excessive platelet aggregation are some of the main mechanisms that have been proposed so far [7–9]. According to other research, the inflammatory reactions to COVID-19 may cause a previously identified atheroma to rupture, which could result in thrombosis and ischemic stroke [10]. However, the rising reports of ischemic strokes linked to COVID-19 infections may be a symptom of this disease's hypercoagulable spectrum. One of the numerous post sequelae problems, post-COVID-19 stroke, has resulted from this and is now progressing.

According to a preliminary retrospective case series investigation from Wuhan, China, acute CVE was the cause in 5.7% of cases with neurological involvement [4]. Following the outbreak, many homes and facilities were quarantined and isolated. As a result, a lot of people spent a lot of time stuck at home or in facilities, which led to inactivity. One of the research projects [11, 12] suggested that this physical inactivity may have increased the risk of a subsequent stroke. 5.88% of patients with new onset CVE were discovered in another recent publication from the same center that examined 221 individuals [13]. Additionally, occurrences of ischemic stroke with no obvious risk factors as the presenting symptom have been described in COVID-19 patients who are not severely unwell [14]. This may bring attention to the variety of COVID-19 ischemic strokes. Additionally, there may have been additional risk factors for the stroke, such as diabetes and high blood pressure. It is unclear, nevertheless, if those traditional risk factors put people at an increased risk of having ischemic episodes after contracting COVID-19. The middle cerebral or posterior cerebral arteries had anterior circulation big artery infarctions in the majority of published cases [15]. Additionally, reports of multifocal strokes in severely unwell individuals are emerging [16]. Therefore, a thorough analysis and understanding of the elevated thrombotic risk in this sensitive population are crucial.

3. Post-COVID-19 stroke and management

To speed up recovery, extensive therapy and a wholistic strategy needed to be used. Rehabilitation is a procedure for solving problems, and it has a strong record of success [17]. It involves identifying the patient's main issues and worries, as well as how they develop and can be resolved. A multidisciplinary team worked together to deliver the appropriate skills to treat and intervene [18] using the holistic biopsychosocial model of illness as a framework [19]. In order to prevent a secondary stroke and other problems, recent research has recommended rehabilitation techniques and treatment for stroke patients during the pandemic [12]. A stroke care model was developed in one study during the COVID-19 epidemic. Its overarching objective was to protect patient outcomes while lowering the risk of COVID-19 exposure for both patients and healthcare professionals [20]. The intensity and extent of their recovery affected the functional gain in terms of regaining independence after the condition. Age was one of the predictor variables that was identified as having a significant impact on functional gain. One such study found that a person's chance of recovery is higher the younger they are. Additionally, the study noted that more limits were seen with longer stays. This was noted as a negative impact of the length of stay on effective ambulation [21]. Hence, to maximize recovery and achieve improved functional outcomes, it is necessary to carefully consider the management and rehabilitation of such a susceptible population.

Treatment and recovery for stroke victims who also have COVID-19 infection are very different from those who do not. According to recent studies, stroke patients with COVID-19 had worse clinical outcomes than stroke patients without COVID-19 [22]. This could be as a result of the various comorbidities that stroke survivors with COVID-19 may have. In addition to the typical clinical symptoms of a stroke patient, a person with COVID-19 infection may also exhibit dyspnea, extreme fatigue, a low endurance tolerance, musculoskeletal abnormalities, and diminished cardiovascular and respiratory functioning. In one study, 51.2% of COVID-19-infected stroke patients died, and the survivors were referred to rehabilitation centers for additional care [23]. In a different study, patients with COVID-19 had higher median National Institutes of Health Stroke Scale (NIHSS) scores than patients without COVID-19. Additionally, stroke patients who had COVID-19 had a greater probability of dying and suffering from severe impairment [24]. This might explain why stroke patients with COVID-19 receive different rehabilitation than stroke patients without

COVID-19. Future research needs to be done to fully understand the long-term risks, manifestations, and the appropriate management for this emerging rehabilitation population.

4. Conclusion

Acute ischemic stroke caused by COVID-19 is regarded as a crippling condition to be worried about. To manage such a fragile population, there are many different treatment approaches and rehabilitation best practices. To assess a patient's rehabilitation needs, a multidisciplinary team approach with a holistic point of view is advised and necessary. To manage such mixed diagnoses efficiently, a team must have goals and move quickly. To prevent and manage the infection that causes strokes, it is critical to have a thorough grasp of the underlying mechanisms. In order to develop a clearer picture of how COVID-19 infection predisposes to stroke and other problems, extreme caution must be used, and further study must be conducted. Future research would benefit from this review.

Acknowledgements

We would like to acknowledge the support of the administration of Qatar Rehabilitation Institute and the Medical Research Center (HMC, Qatar) in encouraging and enabling us to engage in this endeavor.

Conflict of interest

The authors declare no conflict of interest.

Notes/thanks/other declarations

Thanks: The authors wish to acknowledge and thank the entire therapy team and the hospital for supporting in this endeavor.

Acronyms and abbreviations

FIM	functional independence measure
CVE	cerebrovascular events
AIS	acute ischemic stroke

Author details

Thajus Asirvatham[1*], Premraj Isaac Chandran[1] and Ajay Boppana[2]

1 Department of Occupational Therapy, Qatar Rehabilitation Institute, Hamad Medical Corporation, Doha, Qatar

2 Qatar Rehabilitation Institute, Hamad Medical Corporation, Doha, Qatar

*Address all correspondence to: tasirvatham@hamad.qa

IntechOpen

© 2023 The Author(s). Licensee IntechOpen. This chapter is distributed under the terms of the Creative Commons Attribution License (http://creativecommons.org/licenses/by/3.0), which permits unrestricted use, distribution, and reproduction in any medium, provided the original work is properly cited.

References

[1] Joshi RS, Jagdale SS, Bansode SB, Shankar SS, Tellis MB, Pandya VK, et al. Discovery of potential multi-target-directed ligands by targeting host specific SARS-CoV-2 structurally conserved main protease. Journal of Biomolecular Structure & Dynamics. 2021;**39**(9):3099-3114. DOI: 10.1080/07391102.2020.1760137

[2] Kundu D, Selvaraj C, Singh SK, Dubey VK. Identification of new anti-nCoV drug chemical compounds from Indian spices exploiting SARS-CoV-2 main protease as target. Journal of Biomolecular Structure & Dynamics. 2021;**39**(9):3428-3434. DOI: 10.1080/07391102.2020.1763202

[3] Schweickert WD, Pohlman MC, Pohlman AS, Nigos C, Pawlik AJ, Esbrook CL, et al. Early physical and occupational therapy in mechanically ventilated,critically ill patients: A randomized controlled trial. Lancet. 2009;**373**(9678):1874-1882. DOI: 10.1016/S0140-6736(09)60658-9

[4] Mao L, Jin H, Wang M, Hu Y, Chen S, He Q, et al. Neurologic manifestations of hospitalized patients with coronavirus disease 2019 in Wuhan, China. JAMA Neurology. 2020;**77**(6):683-690. DOI: 10.1001/ jamaneurol.2020.1127

[5] Tan Y-K, Goh C, Leow AST, Tambyah PA, Ang A, Yap ES, et al. COVID-19 and ischemic stroke: A systematic review and meta-summary of the literature. Journal of Thrombosis and Thrombolysis. 2020;**50**(3):587-595. DOI: 10.1007/s11239-020-02228-y

[6] Ni W, Yang X, Yang D, Bao J, Li R, Xiao Y, et al. Role of angiotensin-converting enzyme 2 (ACE2) in COVID-19. Critical Care. 2020;**24**:422. DOI: 10.1186/s13054-020-03120-0

[7] Najjar S, Najjar A, Chong DJ, Pramanik BK, Kirsch C, Kuzniecky RI, et al. Central nervous system complications associated with SARS-CoV-2 infection: Integrative concepts of pathophysiology and case reports. Journal of Neuroinflammation. 2020;**17**:231. DOI: 10.1186/s12974-020-01896-0

[8] Spence JD, de Freitas GR, Pettigrew LC, Ay H, Liebeskind DS, Kase CS, et al. Mechanisms of stroke in COVID-19. Cerebrovascular Diseases. 2020;**49**:451-458. DOI: 10.1159/000509581

[9] Gupta A, Madhavan MV, Sehgal K, Nair N, Mahajan S, Sehrawat TS, et al. Extrapulmonary manifestations of COVID-19. Nature Medicine. 2020;**26**:1017-1032. DOI: 10.1038/s41591-020-0968-3

[10] Schonrich G, Raftery MJ, Samstag Y. Devilishly radical NETwork in COVID-19: Oxidative stress, neutrophil extracellular traps (NETs), and T cell suppression. Advanced Biology Regulation. 2020;**77**:100741. DOI: 10.1016/j.jbior.2020.100741

[11] Siegler JE, Heslin ME, Thau L, Smith A, Jovin TG. Falling stroke rates during COVID-19 pandemic at a comprehensive stroke center. Journal of Stroke and Cerebrovascular Diseases. 2020 Aug;**29**(8):104953. DOI: 10.1016/j.jstrokecerebrovasdis.2020.104953

[12] Wang CC, Chao JK, Wang ML, Yang YP, Chien CS, Lai WY, et al. Care for patients with stroke during the COVID-19 pandemic: Physical therapy and rehabilitation suggestions for preventing secondary stroke. Journal of Stroke Cerebrovascular Diseases.

2020;**29**(11):105182. DOI: 10.1016/j.jstrokecerebrovasdis.2020.105182.Epub

[13] Filatov A, Sharma P, Hindi F, Espinosa PS. Neurological complications of coronavirus disease (COVID-19): Encephalopathy. Cureus. 2020;**12**(3):e7352 Available from: https://www.cureus.com/articles/29414-neurological-complications-ofcoronavirus-disease-covid-19-encephalopathy

[14] Diaz-Segarra N, Edmond A, Kunac A, Yonclas P. COVID-19 ischemic strokes as an emerging rehabilitation population: A case series. American Journal of Physical Medicine & Rehabilitation. 2020;**99**(10):876-879. DOI: 10.1097/PHM.0000000000001532

[15] Oxley TJ, Mocco J, Majidi S, et al. Large-vessel stroke as a presenting feature of Covid-19 in the young. The New England Journal of Medicine. 2020;**2020**:e60. DOI: 10.1056/NEJMc2009787

[16] Zhang Y, Xiao M, Zhang S, et al. Coagulopathy and antiphospholipid antibodies in patients with Covid-19. The New England Journal of Medicine. 2020;**2020**. DOI: 10.1056/NEJMc2007575

[17] Wade DT. What is rehabilitation? An empirical investigation leading to an evidence-based description. Clinical Rehabilitation. 2020;**34**(5):571-583. DOI: 10.1177/0269215520905112

[18] Wade D. A Teamwork Approach to Neurological Rehabilitation [Internet]. Oxford Textbook of Neurorehabilitation. Oxford University Press; 2021. Available from: https://oxfordmedicine.com/view/10.1093/med/9780198824954.001.0001/med-9780198824954-chapter-2

[19] Wade DT, Halligan PW. The biopsychosocial model of illness: A model whose time has come. Clinical Rehabilitation. 2017;**31**(8):995-1004. DOI: 10.1177/0269215517709890

[20] Meyer D, Meyer BC, Rapp KS, Modir R, Agrawal K, Hailey L, et al. A stroke care model at an academic, comprehensive stroke center during the 2020 COVID-19 pandemic. Journal of Stroke and Cerebrovascular Diseases. 2020;**29**(8):104927. DOI: 10.1016/j.jstrokecerebrovasdis.2020.104927

[21] Asirvatham T, Abubacker M, Isaac Chandran P, Boppana A, al Salim Abdulla S, Mohammed Saad R. Post-COVID-19 stroke rehabilitation in Qatar: A retrospective, Observational Pilot Study. Qatar Medical Journal. 2022;**28**(1):10. DOI: 10.5339/qmj.2022.10

[22] Sweid A, Hammoud B, Bekelis K, Missios S, Tjoumakaris SI, Gooch MR, et al. Cerebral ischemic and hemorrhagic complications of coronavirus disease 2019. International Journal of Stroke. 2020;**15**(7):733-742. DOI: 10.1177/1747493020937189

[23] Fatima N, Saqqur M, Qamar F, Shaukat S, Shuaib A. Impact of COVID-19 on neurological manifestations: An overviewof stroke presentation in pandemic. Neurological Sciences. 2020;**41**(10):2675-2679. DOI: 10.1007/s10072-020-04637-6 Epub 2020 Aug 6

[24] Ntaios G, Michel P, Georgiopoulos G, Guo Y, Li W, Xiong J, et al. Characteristics and outcomes in patients with COVID-19 and acute ischemic stroke. Stroke. 2020;**51**:e254-e258. DOI: 10.1161/STROKEAHA.120.031208

Chapter 4

Post-COVID-19 and Mental Health

Teodora Safiye, Ardea Milidrag, Said Čekić, Draško Dubljanin, Andreja Kovačević, Milena Zlatanović, Merdin Markišić, Mile Despotović and Medo Gutić

Abstract

Beginning with its emergence in Wuhan, China, in December 2019, severe acute respiratory syndrome coronavirus 2 (SARS-CoV-2), a pandemic that causes COVID-19, has spread and left profound consequences on the lives and health of people around the world. Although most patients who have COVID-19 recover after two to six weeks, research shows that 10–30% of people who have had COVID-19, even with a mild clinical picture, remain with persistent symptoms that have a devastating effect on their quality of life. These symptoms, which most often include fatigue, shortness of breath, chest pain, headache, and cognitive dysfunction, but also others that generally have an impact on everyday functioning, are recognized as a clinical condition called post-COVID syndrome (long COVID). In addition to physical disabilities in people recovering from COVID-19, mental health problems have also been observed, including problems with concentration ("brain fog"), anxiety, depression, sleep disorders, and symptoms of post-traumatic stress disorder (PTSD). In this chapter, we provide a comprehensive review of the current scientific findings identifying post-COVID conditions and their relationship with mental health status.

Keywords: long-term effects of COVID-19, mental health, post-COVID, post-COVID-19 conditions, anxiety, epression

1. Introduction

The emergence of severe acute respiratory syndrome coronavirus 2 (SARS-CoV-2) caused a devastating pandemic. COVID-19, which stands for Coronavirus Disease 2019, is an infectious disease that can affect people of all ages in many ways. Most people infected with SARS-CoV-2 develop mild to moderate disease with viral replication confined mainly to the upper respiratory tract. However, acute respiratory distress syndrome (ARDS) can develop when a virus from the upper respiratory tract spreads to the lungs and produces viral pneumonia and lung damage. When severe, it impairs the body's capacity to maintain vital oxygen levels in the blood, which can result in a number of body system failures and even lead to death [1]. Old age, obesity, and being male are well-established risk factors for severe outcomes of the COVID-19. Various preexisting conditions are also associated with an increased risk. For example, common comorbidities associated with an increased risk of death include hypertension, heart failure, cardiac arrhythmia, diabetes, renal failure, and chronic lung disease [1–3].

The aforementioned infectious disease COVID-19 has rapidly affected mortality worldwide. Globally, till today, there have been 632 million confirmed cases of COVID-19, including 6.5 million deaths, reported to the World Health Organization (WHO) [4].

Although most patients who have COVID-19 recover after two to six weeks, research shows that 10–30% of people who have had COVID-19, even with a mild clinical picture, remain with persistent symptoms that have a devastating effect on their quality of life. These symptoms, which most often include fatigue, shortness of breath, chest pain, headache, and cognitive dysfunction, but also others, which generally have an impact on everyday functioning, are recognized as a clinical condition called post-COVID syndrome (long COVID) [5].

In addition to physical disabilities in people recovering from COVID-19, mental health problems have also been observed, including problems with concentration ("brain fog"), anxiety, depression, sleep disorders, and symptoms of post-traumatic stress disorder (PTSD) [6].

In this chapter, we provide a comprehensive review of the current scientific findings identifying post-COVID conditions and the relationship with mental health status.

2. Post-COVID-19 conditions

Although respiratory symptoms make up the majority of COVID-19's clinical presentation due to the SARS-CoV-2 infection, other conditions like pulmonary (such as pneumonia or dyspnea with exertion), gastrointestinal (such as anorexia or diarrhea), neurological (such as headache, anosmia, or dizziness), or even cardiac ones (such as ischemia, arrhythmias, or myocarditis) may also manifest. It is now well established that nearly a third of patients worldwide will have persistent symptoms for weeks and months, sometimes up to a year after being diagnosed with COVID-19 [7]. These results, particularly for patients who had severe symptoms and spent many weeks in intensive care, are comparable to the recovery from SARS in 2003. But COVID-19 is different because a large portion of those who do not need to be hospitalized seem to relapse, persist, or manifest new symptoms months after the initial infection [8].

When SARS-CoV and MERS-CoV outbreaks occurred in the past, people who recovered from these viral illnesses were left with lingering symptoms like extreme fatigue, a lower quality of life, protracted shortness of breath, and behavioral health issues. These symptoms have put a significant burden on the local health-care systems where the outbreak occurred. Similarly, despite scientific evidence that SARS-CoV-2 replication stops four weeks after the commencement of infection (on the basis of sampling viral isolates from the respiratory tract, not the nasopharyngeal/oropharyngeal sample), a collection of distinct clinical symptoms known as post-COVID-19 syndrome has been reported in a minority of patients who have recovered from COVID-19 caused by SARS-CoV-2 [9]. A meta-analysis including 4828 post-COVID-19 patients showed that symptoms and post-acute sequelae of SARS-CoV-2 can persist for weeks to months after the infection [10].

Persistent symptoms after the COVID-19 illness are called long-term COVID or post-acute sequelae of COVID-19. Some individuals who have contracted the virus that causes COVID-19 may go on to develop post-COVID conditions (PCC) or long COVID as a result of their infection. Long-haul COVID, post-acute COVID-19, post-acute sequelae of SARS CoV-2 infection (PASC), long-term effects of COVID, and chronic COVID are only a few of the terms used to describe post-COVID problems [11].

The hallmark of post-acute COVID-19 syndrome is the continuation of clinical symptoms for longer than four weeks following the beginning of acute symptoms [9]. The term "post-COVID conditions" was created by the Center for Disease Control (CDC) to characterize health issues that last longer than four weeks after getting COVID-19. The following conditions fall under this category: multi-organ COVID-19 effects, impacts of COVID-19 treatment/hospitalization, and extended COVID or persistent post-COVID syndrome (PPCS) [9].

Clinically, "long covid" is characterized by symptoms such as weariness, dyspnea, exhaustion, brain fog, headache, persistent loss of smell or taste, cough, sadness, low fever, palpitations, dizziness, muscle and joint pain, and autonomic dysfunction [9, 12].

The multi-organ effects of COVID-19 include clinical manifestations involving the cardiovascular, pulmonary, renal, and neuropsychiatric organ systems, although the duration of these multi-organ effects is unclear [9, 13].

The long-term "effects of treatment or hospitalization for COVID-19" are similar to other severe infections. These include post-intensive care syndrome (PICS), which consists of impairment of cognition, psychological health, and physical function in an intensive care unit survivor. It can also include muscle weakness, problems with thinking and judgment, and symptoms of PTSD. Many patients with these complications caused by COVID-19 recover over time [9, 14].

In addition to morbidity and mortality in the acute phase, post-acute health problems and consequences have also been recorded in persons who have survived COVID-19. According to the review, up to 80% of patients with COVID-19 continue to complain of health problems after the acute infection and more than 50 side effects have been reported [15]. Post-acute COVID-19 was categorized as follows by Nalbandian et al. based on the severity of symptoms following COVID-19 infection: After the initial acute episode, subacute or persistent COVID-19 symptoms can last up to 12 weeks, and chronic or post-COVID syndrome symptoms start to show up after that. This should not, however, be attributed to a different diagnosis [16].

A large observational cohort study from 38 US hospitals assessed the outcomes of 1250 COVID-19 survivors 60 days after hospital discharge using medical record abstraction and telephone surveys. During the study period, 6.7% of patients died, while 15.1% of patients required readmission. Out of a total of 488 patients who completed the telephone survey, 32.6% of patients reported persistent symptoms including 18.9% with new or worsening symptoms. In this study, 159 individuals reported experiencing cardiopulmonary symptoms (e.g. cough or dyspnea), including 92 who experienced new or worsening symptoms and 65 who experienced irreversible loss of taste or smell. Fifty-eight patients reported new or deteriorating difficulties carrying out their everyday tasks. Among the 195 patients who had jobs prior to being admitted to the hospital, 117 were able to go back to work, while 78 were unable to do so due to continued health issues or job loss. Almost half of all patients (238 of 488) reported being emotionally affected by their health, and 28 sought mental health care after discharge [17].

Similar findings were obtained in studies conducted in Europe. In a population-based prospective cohort study conducted in Spain to determine post-COVID-19 complications and risk factors among patients six months after SARS-CoV-2 infection, in a sample of 484 patients, it was shown that 160 patients (33.1%) experienced at least one post-COVID-19 problem after six months, and 47 of them (29.5%) sought medical help. Hair loss, exhaustion, loss of taste or smell, and headache were the most prevalent long-lasting effects. The complication's risk factors included female gender, age over 35 years, current smoker, and exposure to COVID-19. A third of patients had persistent symptoms compatible with long-term COVID-19 syndrome [18]. In 143 patients who were discharged from the hospital after recovering from acute COVID-19 at a median time of up to 60 days following the onset of symptoms, a post-acute outpatient clinic established in Italy revealed that 87.4% of patients had persistent symptoms. The most frequently reported symptoms were fatigue (53.1%), dyspnea (43.4%), joint pain (27.3%), and chest pain (21.7%), and 55% of patients continued to experience three or more symptoms. In this study, a decline in quality of life was noted in 44.1% of patients [19]. Also, a study conducted in Brazil confirmed the impact of COVID-19 on worsening health-related quality of life and mental health in COVID-19 patients three months after hospital discharge, compared to that before the onset of COVID-19 symptoms [20].

Other studies have reported similar findings. Results of a prospective follow-up study of 110 survivors in the United Kingdom, 8–12 weeks after hospital admission [21], and 277 survivors in Spain, 10–14 weeks after the disease onset [22], as well as survey studies of 100 UK COVID-19 survivors, 4–8 weeks after discharge [23], and 120 patients discharged from a hospital in France, 100 days after admission [24], showed that fatigue, dyspnea, and psychological distress, such as PTSD, anxiety, depression, and loss of concentration and sleep disorders, observed in approximately 30% or more of study participants at follow-up.

3. Post-COVID-19 conditions and mental health

Of the diverse constellation of symptoms that make up post-COVID-19, some are found in the mental health arena. Neurological and psychiatric symptoms include fatigue, weakness after exertion, cognitive complaints, sensorimotor symptoms, headaches, insomnia, depression, and PTSD [25]. The mechanisms involved in post-COVID-19 development and the factors influencing recovery from COVID-19 are still at an early stage. Current hypotheses include psychological factors, inflammatory and immune responses, and physical deconditioning [26, 27].

Human coronaviruses (including SARS-CoV and MERS-CoV) are one of several groups of viruses thought to be potentially neurotrophic. It has been observed from previous outbreaks that respiratory coronaviruses can penetrate the brain and cerebrospinal fluid, permeating the central nervous system in less than a week, and can then be detected in the cerebrospinal fluid [28]. The perturbation of the immune system caused by the infection could cause psychopathology, and psychiatric consequences have also been observed after previous outbreaks of the coronaviruses. The spread of the pandemic caused by the SARS-CoV-2 virus could be associated with psychiatric implications. Cognitive difficulties are symptomatic features of all psychological disorders [16].

In one cohort study examining the cognitive profile after infection with COVID-19, it was found that 34.3% of patients had cognitive complaints after infection with COVID-19. Patients with headache, anosmia, dysgeusia, diarrhea, and those requiring oxygen therapy had lower scores on subtests of memory, attention, and executive function compared to asymptomatic patients. Patients with headache and clinical hypoxia had lower scores in the global cognitive index, while higher scores in anxiety and depression were found in patients with cognitive complaints. Emotional stress, such as anxiety, depression, and insomnia, can play a role in subjective cognitive complaints. These findings emphasize the importance of early detection of anxiety and depression in order to avoid later neuropsychological impairments in patients with COVID-19 [8].

Cognitive impairment with or without fluctuations, including brain fog, which may manifest as difficulty with concentration, memory, receptive language, and/or executive function, has been observed in patients with COVID-19 [29–31]. Post-COVID brain fog in critically ill patients with COVID-19 may develop from mechanisms such as deconditioning or PTSD. However, reports of COVID-19-induced brain fog following mild COVID-19 illness suggest that dysautonomia may also contribute. Finally, long-term cognitive impairment is well recognized in the post-critical phase of the disease, occurring in 20–40% of patients discharged from intensive care units [31–34].

Numerous studies have been published on mental health of people around the world during the COVID-19 pandemic reporting varying rates of mental health problems. Findings from extensive scientific literature indicate that the outbreak of the COVID-19 pandemic increased the prevalence of mental health problems by a massive 25%, worldwide [35].

A large body of evidence suggests that there is a mixed but significant increase in mental health problems among general population [36–40], but also among other specific populations, such as patients with preexisting chronic health conditions [41–43], patients with preexisting severe mental disorders [44–47], and alcohol addicts [48–50]. Also, an increased prevalence of anxiety and depression symptoms was noted in the population of health-care workers during the pandemic [51], with psychological distress and insomnia [52], as well as physical and mental exhaustion and burnout [53–56].

Individuals with COVID-19 experience a range of psychiatric symptoms that persist or occur months after the initial infection [57].

In a study conducted in Italy on a sample of 402 people who recovered from COVID-19, the psychopathological impact of COVID-19 on survivors was examined taking into account the effect of clinical and inflammatory predictors. It showed that one month after hospitalization, a significant proportion of patients self-rated in the psychopathological range: 28% for PTSD, 31% for depression, 42% for anxiety, 20% for symptoms of obsessive-compulsive disorder (OCD), and 40% for insomnia. Approximately 56% of COVID-19 survivors were positive in at least one of the domains assessed for psychiatric sequelae (PTSD, depression, anxiety, insomnia, and obsessive-compulsive symptomatology). Patients with a previously confirmed psychiatric diagnosis showed increased scores on most psychopathological measures [58].

One systematic review included peer-reviewed studies reporting on neuropsychiatric symptoms at post-acute or later time points after COVID-19 infection and in control groups where available. The total number of subjects was 18,917 patients and the average duration of follow-up after recovery from COVID-19 was 77 days. The quality of the studies was mostly moderate. The most common neuropsychiatric symptom was sleeping disturbance (total prevalence = 27.4%), followed by fatigue (24.4%), objective cognitive impairment (20.2%), anxiety (19.1%), and PTSD (15.7%). Two studies in the review compared COVID-19 patients with controls and found that COVID-19 patients had higher levels of mental health symptoms. Based on hospitalization status, infection severity, or length of follow-up, there was no difference in the prevalence of mental health problems among COVID-19 patients across the studies in the review [59].

There are numerous obstacles in the literature to date regarding the mental health aspects of the post-COVID-19 condition, including the dearth of studies with active control groups for attributing COVID-19 illness symptoms, the lack of consensus on the term "post-COVID-19 condition," and diverse participant selection criteria [60].

In addition to seriously affecting mental health and well-being of people around the world, the COVID-19 pandemic has also raised concerns about increased suicidal behavior. Factors that may increase suicidal risk during a pandemic, especially in vulnerable groups (such as people with a previous history of psychiatric disorder, people over 65, people who have already attempted suicide, COVID-19 frontline health-care workers, people infected with the coronavirus, and people who are recovering from COVID-19, as well as people whose family member or friend died of COVID-19), are social isolation; anxiety; fear of infection; prolonged stress; job insecurity and unemployment; and access to food, education, and health care in the non-COVID system [61, 62].

The few available studies on the mental status of patients with COVID-19 provide us with preliminary information about how psychiatric symptoms associated with COVID-19 develop and change. During the hospital stay, a significantly high proportion of patients reported depression (60.2%), anxiety (55.3%) [63], and PTSD (96.2%) [64]. Liu et al. [65] found that the prevalence rate of clinically significant depression, anxiety, and PTSD symptoms in COVID-19 patients after hospital discharge was 19%, 10.4%, and 12.4%, which is a significant drop compared to the findings of the previously mentioned studies. The adverse effects of COVID-19 on mental health are evident after discharge from hospital, with sleep difficulties highlighted as a central issue. Also, Liu et al. pointed out that perceived discrimination is a central predictor of mental illness and that preventing and addressing the social stigma associated with COVID-19 can be crucial for improving the mental health of recovered patients [65].

High rates of mental health problems, especially anxiety, depression, suicidal behavior, and PTSD, have been reported in general population and after previous coronavirus epidemics, regardless of infectious status [66, 67]. One study conducted in South Korea on a sample of patients quarantined for suspected or confirmed MERS-CoV found that 40% of patients were given a psychiatric diagnosis while in the hospital and that 70.8% of confirmed patients who survived the illness displayed psychiatric symptoms, including hallucinations and psychosis. None of the individuals who had MERS-CoV that was suspected but not yet confirmed displayed any symptoms suggesting a possible viral mechanism underlying psychiatric disorders, a dose-response effect, or a greater psychological effect of receiving a confirmed diagnosis of respiratory disease [68]. A study involving 90 cases with SARS-CoV similarly showed high levels of psychological distress with 59% diagnosed with psychiatric disorders and a continued prevalence of 33% at thirty-month follow-up. The severity of psychological symptoms was found to be related to disease severity and functional impairment [69, 70].

Several long-term health complications in previous coronavirus infections are well documented. A review that included 34 studies and aimed to assess physical and mental health after problems with COVID-19, with a follow-up period longer than one month after discharge or after the onset of symptoms, showed that the most frequently reported mental health problems were anxiety (ranging from 6.5% to 63%), depression (4–31%), and PTSD (12.1–46.9%). Patients and people admitted to critical care noted higher levels of exhaustion, pain, anxiety, and depression. Up to three months following COVID-19, a general decline in quality of life was observed.

Up to three months following COVID-19, various physical and mental health issues were present, according to this review. Findings indicate the necessity of thorough evaluation and rehabilitation following COVID-19 to improve the quality of life [71].

Sleep problems are another prominent post-COVID-19 mental health problem, especially insomnia, which has been observed in both the acute and chronic stages of the disease [24, 72–74]. Other studies have also suggested that sleep problems are a central complication perceived among COVID-19 survivors [65, 75, 76]. Sleep difficulties, anxiety, and depression were present in approximately one-quarter of patients at six-month follow-up after acute COVID-19 in a study conducted in China [77].

Clinically significant depression and anxiety have been reported in approximately 30–40% of patients following COVID-19, similar to patients with previous severe SARS, starting in 2002, and MERS, starting in 2012 [78–81]. Clinically significant PTSD symptoms have been reported in approximately 30% of COVID-19 patients requiring hospitalization and may occur early during acute infection or months later [58, 81].

An analysis of a large-scale data set that included 62,354 patients who survived COVID-19 from 54 health-care organizations in the United States estimated that between days 14 and 90 following diagnosis, there were 18.1% first-time and recurrent cases of psychiatric disorder. More significantly, it revealed that among a subset of 44,759 patients without a history of psychiatric illness, the estimated overall probability of developing a new psychiatric illness within 90 days of a COVID-19 diagnosis was 5.8% (anxiety disorder = 4.7%; mood disorder = 2%; insomnia = 1.9%; dementia (among those under 65 years) = 1.6%). All these values were significantly higher than in the corresponding control cohorts of patients diagnosed with influenza and other respiratory infections. Survivors of COVID-19 appear to be at increased risk for psychiatric sequelae, and a psychiatric diagnosis may be an independent risk factor for COVID-19 [82].

The prevalence of mental health issues varies significantly across studies, which may be a result of variations in the measures used to assess these outcomes as well as regional variations in the influence of cultural or spiritual beliefs on attempts to manage the psychological impact of coronavirus disease [83].

Although higher rates of psychiatric symptoms can be expected in the general population after a pandemic due to exposure to traumatic life events such as death of friends and relatives, loss of income, fear, and general psychological distress, within this group there may also be individuals whose cognitive and psychological disorders are directly related with brain changes caused by the coronavirus. For this reason, the question can be raised as to how the mentioned group will respond to standard treatment, for example, antidepressants, anxiolytics, and cognitive therapies [30].

Treatments such as cognitive-behavioral psychotherapy (CBT) are recommended for various psychiatric manifestations of the post-COVID condition, such as chronic fatigue syndrome [84]. However, face-to-face cognitive-behavioral psychotherapy is a time-intensive treatment and the question is how applicable it is during the pandemic due to various government restrictions that include physical and social distancing to prevent further spread of the virus [85]. Despite this, new modern ways of digital communication can enable effective support in the form of rehabilitation services provided through information and communication technologies, especially in the situation of an infectious disease pandemic and among COVID-19 survivors [86–88]. Computer-based interventions target improvement of physical and emotional functioning in patients with chronic pain and functional somatic syndromes [89]. Internet-delivered cognitive behavioral therapy (I-CBT) has been reported to be an effective and efficient treatment for psychiatric problems and musculoskeletal symptoms, compared to waiting lists or usual care settings, and may be equivalent to traditional (face-to-face) forms of provision [90–92].

Therefore, telehealth (telerehabilitation and telepsychiatry) could be considered as a follow-up treatment in an effort to prevent long-term physical and mental health complications in post-COVID-19 patients [93].

4. Mental health issues in the post-COVID-19 era

Evidence suggests that there is a significant increase in mental health problems among general population and vulnerable groups. Previous major public health crises have shown that more than half of the population developed mental health problems and needed mental health intervention [94].

In the post-pandemic era, it may be difficult to identify mental disorders etiologically related to COVID-19 (e.g. cytokine storm anxiety) due to the lack of specific diagnostic or screening tools. Due to limited scientific understanding of the link between COVID-19 and mental health so far, post-pandemic preparedness is difficult. Clinicians, researchers, and policymakers are expected to be prepared for these mental health issues in terms of assessment, interventions, and models of care in the post-pandemic era [94].

Given the global scale of the pandemic, it is clear that health-care needs for patients affected by the effects of COVID-19 will continue to grow for the foreseeable future. Meeting this challenge will require leveraging existing and developing new health-care models and interdisciplinary collaboration to improve both the physical and mental health of COVID-19 survivors in the long term [95].

Data reporting mental health consequences of coronavirus infection, especially long-term, are needed to improve treatment, mental health-care planning, and preventive measures during the COVID-19 pandemic. It is necessary to conduct active medical monitoring of patients post-COVID-19, and since post-COVID-19 physical and mental health problems that can reduce the quality of life can persist for three months or longer after the illness, early examination and comprehensive planning of rehabilitation of patients may be needed to effectively prevent and manage post-COVID-19 complications, which could reduce economic and clinical health consequences and prevent long-term disability [96].

5. Conclusions

SARS-CoV-2 outbreak can be considered a unique mental health disaster. Most studies have reported psychological and neuropsychological problems (anxiety and depression, PTSD, sleep problems, and cognitive problems) post-COVID-19, even in people without previously diagnosed mental health problems. PTSD is the most prevalent long-term post-COVID psychiatric condition, followed by depression and anxiety disorders.

Aside from causing physical illness, SARS-CoV-2 also has long-term negative effects on mental health. The crucial question of what causes these mental health issues cannot be precisely answered based on the information now available. They could result from the virus's direct effects on the brain and central nervous system, but they could also be brought on by the stress of being hospitalized with a disease that is poorly understood in the midst of widespread social anxiety or by experiences like witnessing the deaths of other patients in the hospital, or family members. It is quite reasonable to conclude that psychological symptoms resulting from infection with the coronavirus last much longer than the physical symptoms of the disease.

The results of conducted scientific research on the connection between the post-COVID-19 state and mental health emphasize the need to increase the readiness and competence of health workers in detecting and managing the psychological consequences of future comparable outbreaks of infectious diseases. It is clear that care for patients with COVID-19 does not end at hospital discharge, and currently, health-care professionals caring for acute COVID-19 survivors have a key role in recognizing, carefully documenting, investigating, and managing ongoing or new symptoms, as well as monitoring of organ-specific complications that developed during an acute illness.

Ultimately, additional research is needed regarding the long-term impact of COVID-19 on mental health.

Acknowledgements

The authors acknowledge all those who, through their good deeds or misdeeds, contributed to the authors' scientific success.

Author details

Teodora Safiye[1*], Ardea Milidrag[1], Said Čekić[2], Draško Dubljanin[1,3], Andreja Kovačević[1,4], Milena Zlatanović[1,5], Merdin Markišić[2], Mile Despotović[5] and Medo Gutić[1,6]

1 Faculty of Medical Sciences, University of Kragujevac, Kragujevac, Serbia

2 Faculty of Pharmacy and Health, University of Travnik, Travnik, Bosnia and Herzegovina

3 Department of Pulmonology, University Clinical Hospital Center Zvezdara, Belgrade, Serbia

4 Department of Cardio-Pulmonary Rehabilitation, Institute for Rehabilitation Belgrade, Belgrade, Serbia

5 Department Ćuprija, Academy of Educational and Medical Vocational Studies Kruševac, Serbia

6 Public Health Institution Health Center "Dr Branko Zogović", Plav, Montenegro

*Address all correspondence to: teodoras0306@gmail.com

IntechOpen

© 2023 The Author(s). Licensee IntechOpen. This chapter is distributed under the terms of the Creative Commons Attribution License (http://creativecommons.org/licenses/by/3.0), which permits unrestricted use, distribution, and reproduction in any medium, provided the original work is properly cited.

References

[1] Lamers MM, Haagmans BL. SARS-CoV-2 pathogenesis. Nature Reviews Microbiology. 2022;**20**:270-284. DOI: 10.1038/s41579-022-00713-0

[2] Karagiannidis C, Mostert C, Hentschker C, Voshaar T, Malzahn J, Schillinger G, et al. Case characteristics, resource utilization and outcomes of 10,021 patients with COVID-19 admitted to 920 German hospitals: An observational study. The Lancet Respiratory Medicine. 2020;**8**:853-862. DOI: 10.1016/S2213-2600(20)30316-7

[3] Williamson EJ, Walker AJ, Bhaskaran K, Bacon S, Bates C, Morton CE, et al. Factors associated with death associated with COVID 19 using OpenSAFELY. Nature. 2020;**584**:430-436. DOI: 10.1038/s41586-020-2521-4

[4] WHO. Weekly Epidemiological Update on COVID-19—16 November 2022. 2022. Available from: https://www.who.int/publications/m/item/weekly-epidemiological-update-on-covid-19---16-november-2022. [Accessed: November 18, 2022]

[5] Garg M, Maralakunte M, Garg S, Dhooria S, Sehgal I, Bhalla AS, et al. The conundrum of 'Long-COVID-19': A narrative review. International Journal of General Medicine. 2021;**14**:2491-2506. DOI: 10.2147/IJGM.S316708

[6] Krishnan K, Lin Y, Prewitt KM, Potter DA. Multidisciplinary approach to brain fog and related persisting symptoms post COVID-19. Journal of Health Service Psychology. 2022;**48**:31-38. DOI: 10.1007/s42843-022-00056-7

[7] Taquet M, Geddes JR, Husain M, Luciano S, Harrison PJ. 6-month neurological and psychiatric outcomes in 236 379 survivors of COVID-19: A retrospective cohort study using electronic health records. Lancet Psychiatry. 2021;**8**:416-427. DOI: 10.1016/S2215-0366(21)00084-5

[8] Almeria M, Cejudo JC, Sotoca J, Deus J, Krupinski J. Cognitive profile following COVID-19 infection: Clinical predictors leading to neuropsychological impairment. Brain, Behavior, and Immunity—Health. 2020;**9**:100163. DOI: 10.1016/j.bbih.2020.100163

[9] Chippa V, Aleem A, Anjum F. Post acute coronavirus (COVID-19) syndrome. In: StatPearls [Internet]. Treasure Island (FL): StatPearls Publishing. p. 2022

[10] Malik P, Patel K, Pinto C, Jaiswal R, Tirupathi R, Pillai S, et al. Post-acute COVID-19 syndrome (PCS) and health-related quality of life (HRQoL)—A systematic review and meta-analysis. Journal of Medical Virology. 2022;**94**:253-262. DOI: 10.1002/jmv.27309

[11] CDC. Long COVID or Post-COVID Conditions. Available from: https://www.cdc.gov/coronavirus/2019-ncov/long-term-effects/index.html. [Accessed: January 10, 2022]

[12] Joli J, Buck P, Zipfel S, Stengel A. Post-COVID-19 fatigue: A systematic review. Frontiers in Psychiatry. 2022;**13**:947973. DOI: 10.3389/fpsyt.2022.947973

[13] Zaim S, Chong JH, Sankaranarayanan V, Harky A. COVID-19 and multiorgan response. Current Problems in Cardiology. 2020;**45**:100618. DOI: 10.1016/j.cpcardiol.2020.100618

[14] Rawal G, Yadav S, Kumar R. Post-intensive care syndrome: An overview. Journal of Translational Medicine. 2017;**5**:90-92. DOI: 10.1515/jtim-2016-0016

[15] Lopez-Leon S, Wegman-Ostrosky T, Perelman C, Sepulveda R, Rebolledo PA, Cuapio A, et al. More than 50 long-term effects of COVID-19: A systematic review and meta-analysis. Scientific Reports. 2021;**11**:16144. DOI: 10.1038/s41598-021-95565-8

[16] Nalbandian A, Sehgal K, Gupta A, Madhavan MV, McGroder C, Stevens JS, et al. Post-acute COVID-19 syndrome. Nature Medicine. 2021;**27**:601-615. DOI: 10.1038/s41591-021-01283-z

[17] Chopra V, Flanders SA, O'Malley M, Malani AN, Prescott HC. Sixty-day outcomes among patients hospitalized with COVID-19. Annals of Internal Medicine. 2021;**174**:576-578. DOI: 10.7326/M20-5661

[18] Domènech-Montoliu S, Puig-Barberà J, Pac-Sa MR, Vidal-Utrillas P, Latorre-Poveda M, Del Rio-González A, et al. Complications post-COVID-19 and risk factors among patients after six months of and SARS-CoV-2 infection: A population-based prospective cohort study. Epidemiologia. 2022;**3**:49-67. DOI: 10.3390/epidemiologia3010006

[19] Carfì A, Bernabei R, Landi F. Gemelli against COVID-19 post-acute care study group. Persistent symptoms in patients after acute COVID-19. Journal of the American Medical Association. 2020;**324**:603-605. DOI: 10.1001/jama.2020.12603

[20] Todt BC, Szlejf C, Duim E, Linhares AOM, Kogiso D, Varela G, et al. Clinical outcomes and quality of life of COVID-19 survivors: A follow-up of 3 months post hospital discharge. Respiratory Medicine. 2021;**184**:106453. DOI: 10.1016/j.rmed.2021.106453

[21] Arnold DT, Hamilton FW, Milne A, Morley AJ, Viner J, Attwood M, et al. Patient outcomes after hospitalization with COVID-19 and implications for follow-up: Results from a prospective UK cohort. Thorax. 2021;**76**:399-401. DOI: 10.1136/thoraxjnl-2020-216086

[22] Moreno-Pérez O, Merino E, Leon-Ramirez JM, Andres M, Ramos JM, Arenas-Jiménez J, et al. Post-acute COVID-19 syndrome. Incidence and risk factors: A Mediterranean cohort study. Journal of Infection. 2021;**82**:378-383. DOI: 10.1016/j.jinf.2021.01.004

[23] Halpin SJ, McIvor C, Whyatt G, Adams A, Harvey O, McLean L, et al. Postdischarge symptoms and rehabilitation needs in survivors of COVID-19 infection: A cross-sectional evaluation. Journal of Medical Virology. 2021;**93**:1013-1022. DOI: 10.1002/jmv.26368

[24] Garrigues E, Janvier P, Kherabi Y, Le Bot A, Hamon A, Gouze H, et al. Post-discharge persistent symptoms and health-related quality of life after hospitalization for COVID-19. Journal of Infection. 2020;**81**:e4-e6. DOI: 10.1016/j.jinf.2020.08.029

[25] Pappa S, Barmparessou Z, Athanasiou N, Sakka E, Eleftheriou K, Patrinos S, et al. Depression, insomnia and post-traumatic stress disorder in COVID-19 survivors: Role of gender and impact on quality of life. Journal of Personalized Medicine. 2022;**12**:486. DOI: 10.3390/jpm12030486

[26] Deng J, Zhou F, Hou W, Silver Z, Wong CY, Chang O, et al. The prevalence of depression, anxiety, and sleep disturbances in COVID-19 patients: A meta-analysis. Annals of the New York

Academy of Sciences. 2021;**1486**:90-111. DOI: 10.1111/nyas.14506

[27] Calabrese LH. Cytokine storm and the prospects for immunotherapy with COVID-19. Cleveland Clinic Journal of Medicine. 2020;**87**:389-393. DOI: 10.3949/ccjm.87a.ccc008

[28] Bohmwald K, Gálvez NMS, Ríos M, Kalergis AM. Neurologic alterations due to respiratory virus infections. Frontiers in Cellular Neuroscience. 2018;**12**:386. DOI: 10.3389/fncel.2018.00386

[29] Heneka MT, Golenbock D, Latz E, Morgan D, Brown R. Immediate and long-term consequences of COVID-19 infections for the development of neurological disease. Alzheimer's Research & Therapy. 2020;**12**:69. DOI: 10.1186/s13195-020-00640-3

[30] Ritchie K, Chan D, Watermeyer T. The cognitive consequences of the COVID-19 epidemic: Collateral damage? Brain Communications. 2020;**2**:fcaa069. DOI: 10.1093/braincomms/fcaa069

[31] Kaseda ET, Levine AJ. Post-traumatic stress disorder: A differential diagnostic consideration for COVID-19 survivors. The Clinical Neuropsychologist. 2020;**34**:1498-1514. DOI: 10.1080/13854046.2020.1811894

[32] Novak P. Post COVID-19 syndrome associated with orthostatic cerebral hypoperfusion syndrome, small fiber neuropathy and benefit of immunotherapy: A case report. eNeurologicalSci. 2020;**21**:100276. DOI: 10.1016/j.ensci.2020.100276

[33] Miglis MG, Goodman BP, Chémali KR, Stiles L. Re: 'Post-COVID-19 chronic symptoms' by Davido et al. Clinical Microbiology and Infection. 2021;**27**:494. DOI: 10.1016/j.cmi.2020.08.028

[34] Sakusic A, Rabinstein AA. Cognitive outcomes after critical illness. Current Opinion in Critical Care. 2018;**24**:410-414. DOI: 10.1097/MCC.0000000000000527

[35] Safiye T, Gutić M, Milidrag A, Zlatanović M, Radmanović B. The impact of COVID-19 on mental health: The protective role of resilience and capacity for mentalizing. In: Marques A, Gaspar de Matos M, Sarmento H, editors. Mental Health – Preventive Strategies. London: IntechOpen; 2022. DOI: 10.5772/intechopen.106161

[36] Salari N, Hosseinian-Far A, Jalali R, Vaisi-Raygani A, Rasoulpoor S, Mohammadi M, et al. Prevalence of stress, anxiety, depression among the general population during the COVID-19 pandemic: A systematic review and meta-analysis. Globalization and Health. 2020;**16**:57. DOI: 10.1186/s12992-020-00589-w

[37] Vujčić I, Safiye T, Milikić B, Popović E, Dubljanin D, Dubljanin E, et al. Coronavirus disease 2019 (COVID-19) epidemic and mental health status in the general adult population of Serbia: A cross-sectional study. International Journal of Environmental Research and Public Health. 2021;**18**:1957. DOI: 10.3390/ijerph18041957

[38] Qiu J, Shen B, Zhao M, Wang Z, Xie B, Xu Y. A nationwide survey of psychological distress among Chinese people in the COVID-19 epidemic: Implications and policy recommendations. General Psychiatry. 2020;**33**:e100213. DOI: 10.1136/gpsych-2020-100213

[39] Wu M, Xu W, Yao Y, Zhang L, Guo L, Fan J, et al. Mental health status of students' parents during COVID-19 pandemic and its influence factors. General Psychiatry. 2020;**33**:e100250. DOI: 10.1136/gpsych-2020-100250

[40] Safiye T, Vukčević B. Dimensions of general psychological distress and age as the predictors of procrastination in university students. Psihološka istraživanja. 2020;**24**:187-200. DOI: 10.5937/PSISTRA23-27810

[41] Sayeed A, Kundu S, Al Banna MH, Christopher E, Hasan MT, Begum MR, et al. Mental health outcomes of adults with comorbidity and chronic diseases during the COVID-19 pandemic: A matched case-control study. Psychiatria Danubina. 2020;**32**:491-498. DOI: 10.24869/psyd.2020.491

[42] Dobler CL, Krüger B, Strahler J, Weyh C, Gebhardt K, Tello K, et al. Physical activity and mental health of patients with pulmonary hypertension during the COVID-19 pandemic. Journal of Clinical Medicine. 2020;**9**:4023. DOI: 10.3390/jcm9124023

[43] Xia Y, Kou L, Zhang G, Han C, Hu J, Wan F, et al. Investigation on sleep and mental health of patients with Parkinson's disease during the coronavirus disease 2019 pandemic. Sleep Medicine. 2020;**75**:428-433. DOI: 10.1016/j.sleep.2020.09.011

[44] Pinkham AE, Ackerman RA, Depp CA, Harvey PD, Moore RC. COVID-19-related psychological distress and engagement in preventative behaviors among individuals with severe mental illnesses. NPJ Schizophrenia. 2021;**7**:7. DOI: 10.1038/s41537-021-00136-5

[45] Karantonis JA, Rossell SL, Berk M, Van Rheenen TE. The mental health and lifestyle impacts of COVID-19 on bipolar disorder. Journal of Affective Disorders. 2021;**282**:442-447. DOI: 10.1016/j.jad.2020.12.186

[46] Santo F, González-Blanco L, García-Álvarez L, la Fuente-Tomás L, Moya-Lacasa C, Paniagua G, et al. COVID-19 lockdown in people with severe mental disorders in Spain: Do they have a specific psychological reaction? European Neuropsychopharmacology. 2020;**40**:S475-S476. DOI: 10.1016/j.euroneuro.2020.09.618

[47] Yocum AK, Zhai Y, McInnis MG, Han P. Covid-19 pandemic and lockdown impacts: A description in a longitudinal study of bipolar disorder. Journal of Affective Disorders. 2021;**282**:1226-1233. DOI: 10.1016/j.jad.2021.01.028

[48] Barać S, Gutić M, Vukčević B, Safiye T, Radmanović B, Đorđić M, et al. Depression, anxiety and stress among alcohol addicts. Medicinski časopis. 2022;**56**:13-27. DOI: 10.5937/mckg56-35057

[49] Avery AR, Tsang S, Seto EYW, Duncan GE. Stress, anxiety, and change in alcohol use during the COVID-19 pandemic: Findings among adult twin pairs. Frontiers in Psychiatry. 2020;**11**:571084. DOI: 10.3389/fpsyt.2020.571084

[50] Barać S, Vukčević B, Gutić M, Đorđić M, Safiye T. Stress and life satisfaction among alcohol addicts. Medicinski časopis. 2021;**55**:119-130. DOI: 10.5937/mckg55-35483

[51] Sahebi A, Nejati-Zarnaqi B, Moayedi S, Yousefi K, Torres M, Golitaleb M. The prevalence of anxiety and depression among healthcare workers during the COVID-19 pandemic: An umbrella review of meta-analyses. Progress in Neuro-Psychopharmacology & Biological Psychiatry. 2021;**107**:110247. DOI: 10.1016/j.pnpbp.2021.110247

[52] Lai J, Ma S, Wang Y, Cai Z, Hu J, Wei N, et al. Factors associated with mental health outcomes among health-care workers exposed to coronavirus

disease 2019. JAMA Network Open. 2020;**3**:e203976. DOI: 10.1001/jamanetworkopen.2020.3976

[53] Ulfa M, Azuma M, Steiner A. Burnout status of healthcare workers in the world during the peak period of the COVID-19 pandemic. Frontiers in Psychology. 2022;**13**:952783. DOI: 10.3389/fpsyg.2022.952783

[54] Safiye T, Vukčević B, Gutić M, Milidrag A, Dubljanin D, Dubljanin J, et al. Resilience, mentalizing and burnout syndrome among healthcare workers during the COVID-19 pandemic in Serbia. International Journal of Environmental Research and Public Health. 2022;**19**:6577. DOI: 10.3390/ijerph19116577

[55] Stone KW, Kintziger KW, Jagger MA, Horney JA. Public health workforce burnout in the COVID-19 response in the U.S. International Journal of Environmental Research and Public Health. 2021;**18**:4369. DOI: 10.3390/ijerph18084369

[56] Safiye T, Vukčević B, Čabarkapa M. Resilience as a moderator in the relationship between burnout and subjective well-being among medical workers in Serbia during the COVID-19 pandemic. Vojnosanitetski Pregled. 2021;**78**:1207-1213. DOI: 10.2298/VSP210517070S

[57] Postolache TT, Benros ME, Brenner LA. Targetable biological mechanisms implicated in emergent psychiatric conditions associated with SARS-CoV-2 infection. JAMA Psychiatry. 2021;**78**:353-354. DOI: 10.1001/jamapsychiatry.2020.2795

[58] Mazza MG, De Lorenzo R, Conte C, Poletti S, Vai B, Bollettini I, et al. Anxiety and depression in COVID-19 survivors: Role of inflammatory and clinical predictors. Brain, Behavior, and Immunity. 2020;**89**:594-600. DOI: 10.1016/j.bbi.2020.07.037

[59] Badenoch JB, Rengasamy ER, Watson C, Jansen K, Chakraborty S, Sundaram RD, et al. Persistent neuropsychiatric symptoms after COVID-19: A systematic review and meta-analysis. Brain. Communications. 2021;**4**:fcab297. DOI: 10.1093/braincomms/fcab297

[60] WHO. Mental Health and COVID-19: Early Evidence of the Pandemic's Impact: Scientific Brief, 2 March 2022. 2022. Available from: https://www.who.int/publications/i/item/WHO-2019-nCoV-Sci_Brief-Mental_health-2022.1. [Accessed: March 06, 2022]

[61] Stašević-Karličić I, Đorđević V, Dutina A, Stašević M, Janjić V, Ignjatović-Ristić D, et al. The impact of COVID-19 pandemic on suicide attempts in the republic of Serbia. Srpski Arhiv Za Celokupno Lekarstvo. 2021;**149**:455-460. DOI: 10.2298/SARH210506053S

[62] Steeg S, John A, Gunnell DJ, Kapur N, Dekel D, Schmidt L, et al. The impact of the COVID-19 pandemic on presentations to health services following self-harm: Systematic review. The British Journal of Psychiatry. 2022;**221**:603-612. DOI: 10.1192/bjp.2022.79

[63] Guo Q, Zheng Y, Shi J, Wang J, Li G, Li C, et al. Immediate psychological distress in quarantined patients with COVID-19 and its association with peripheral inflammation: A mixed-method study. Brain, Behavior, and Immunity. 2020;**88**:17-27. DOI: 10.1016/j.bbi.2020.05.038

[64] Bo HX, Li W, Yang Y, Wang Y, Zhang Q, Cheung T, et al. Posttraumatic stress symptoms and attitude toward crisis mental health services among clinically

stable patients with COVID-19 in China. Psychological Medicine. 2021;**51**:1052-1053. DOI: 10.1017/S0033291720000999

[65] Liu D, Baumeister RF, Veilleux JC, Chen C, Liu W, Yue Y, et al. Risk factors associated with mental illness in hospital discharged patients infected with COVID-19 in Wuhan. China. Psychiatry Research. 2020;**292**:113297. DOI: 10.1016/j.psychres.2020.113297

[66] Jeong H, Yim HW, Song YJ, Ki M, Min JA, Cho J, et al. Mental health status of people isolated due to Middle East respiratory syndrome. Epidemiology and Health. 2016;**38**:e2016048. DOI: 10.4178/epih.e2016048

[67] Du L, Zhao J, Shi Y, Xi Y, Zheng GG, Yi Y, et al. A report of 4 cases of severe acute respiratory syndrome patients with suicidal tendencies. Academic Journal of Second Military Medical University. 2003;**24**:636-637

[68] Kim HC, Yoo SY, Lee BH, Lee SH, Shin HS. Psychiatric findings in suspected and confirmed Middle East respiratory syndrome patients quarantined in hospital: A retrospective chart analysis. Psychiatry Investigation. 2018;**15**:355-360. DOI: 10.30773/pi.2017.10.25.1

[69] Mak IW, Chu CM, Pan PC, Yiu MG, Chan VL. Long-term psychiatric morbidities among SARS survivors. General Hospital Psychiatry. 2009;**31**:318-326. DOI: 10.1016/j.genhosppsych.2009.03.001

[70] Wing YK, Leung CM. Mental health impact of severe acute respiratory syndrome: A prospective study. Hong Kong Medical Journal. 2012;**18**(Suppl. 3):24-27

[71] Shanbehzadeh S, Tavahomi M, Zanjari N, Ebrahimi-Takamjani I, Amiri-Arimi S. Physical and mental health complications post-COVID-19: Scoping review. Journal of Psychosomatic Research. 2021;**147**:110525. DOI: 10.1016/j .jpsychores.2021.110525

[72] Daher A, Balfanz P, Cornelissen C, Müller A, Bergs I, Marx N, et al. Follow-up of patients with severe coronavirus disease 2019 (COVID-19): Pulmonary and extrapulmonary disease sequelae. Respiratory Medicine. 2020;**174**:106197. DOI: 10.1016/j.rmed.2020.106197

[73] Xiong Q, Xu M, Li J, Liu Y, Zhang J, Xu Y, et al. Clinical sequelae of COVID-19 survivors in Wuhan, China: A single-center longitudinal study. Clinical Microbiology and Infection. 2021;**27**:89-95. DOI: 10.1016/j.cmi.2020.09.023

[74] Hao F, Tam W, Hu X, Tan W, Jiang L, Jiang X, et al. A quantitative and qualitative study on the neuropsychiatric sequelae of acutely ill COVID-19 inpatients in isolation facilities. Translational Psychiatry. 2020;**10**:355. DOI: 10.1038/s41398-020-01039-2

[75] Chen KY, Li T, Gong FH, Zhang JS, Li XK. Predictors of health-related quality of life and influencing factors for COVID-19 patients, a follow-up at one month. Frontiers in Psychiatry. 2020;**11**:668. DOI: 10.3389/fpsyt.2020.00668

[76] Wu C, Hu X, Song J, Yang D, Xu J, Cheng K, et al. Mental health status and related influencing factors of COVID-19 survivors in Wuhan. China. Clinical and Translational Medicine. 2020;**10**:e52. DOI: 10.1002/ctm2.52

[77] Huang C, Huang L, Wang Y, Li X, Ren L, Gu X, et al. 6-month consequences of COVID-19 in patients discharged from hospital: A cohort study. Lancet. 2021;**397**:220-232. DOI: 10.1016/S0140-6736(20)32656-8

[78] Lam MH, Wing YK, Yu MW, Leung CM, Ma RC, Kong AP, et al. Mental morbidities and chronic fatigue in severe acute respiratory syndrome survivors: Long-term follow-up. Archives of Internal Medicine. 2009;**169**:2142-2147. DOI: 10.1001/archinternmed.2009.384

[79] Lee SH, Shin HS, Park HY, Kim JL, Lee JJ, Lee H, et al. Depression as a mediator of chronic fatigue and post-traumatic stress symptoms in Middle East respiratory syndrome survivors. Psychiatry Investigation. 2019;**16**:59-64. DOI: 10.30773/pi.2018.10.22.3

[80] Lee AM, Wong JG, McAlonan GM, Cheung V, Cheung C, Sham PC, et al. Stress and psychological distress among SARS survivors 1 year after the outbreak. Canadian Journal of Psychiatry. 2007;**52**:233-240. DOI: 10.1177/070674370705200405

[81] Rogers JP, Chesney E, Oliver D, Pollak TA, McGuire P, Fusar-Poli P, et al. Psychiatric and neuropsychiatric presentations associated with severe coronavirus infections: A systematic review and meta-analysis with comparison to the COVID-19 pandemic. Lancet Psychiatry. 2020;**7**:611-627. DOI: 10.1016/S2215-0366(20)30203-0

[82] Taquet M, Luciano S, Geddes JR, Harrison PJ. Bidirectional associations between COVID-19 and psychiatric disorder: Retrospective cohort studies of 62 354 COVID-19 cases in the USA. Lancet Psychiatry. 2021;**8**:130-140. DOI: 10.1016/S2215-0366(20)30462-4

[83] Wang C, Chudzicka-Czupała A, Tee ML, Núñez MIL, Tripp C, Fardin MA, et al. A chain mediation model on COVID-19 symptoms and mental health outcomes in Americans, Asians and Europeans. Scientific Reports. 2021;**11**:6481. DOI: 10.1038/s41598-021-85943-7

[84] Castell BD, Kazantzis N, Moss-Morris RE. Cognitive behavioral therapy and graded exercise for chronic fatigue syndrome: A meta-analysis. Clinical Psychology: Science and Practice. 2011;**18**:311-324. DOI: 10.1111/j.1468-2850.2011.01262.x

[85] Čabarkapa M, Safiye T, Gutić M. Psychosocial stress and risk assessment during the COVID-19 pandemic: Some preliminary thoughts. International Journal of Population Studies. 2022;**8**:1-5. DOI: 10.18063/ijps.v8i2.1335

[86] Salawu A, Green A, Crooks MG, Brixey N, Ross DH, Sivan M. A proposal for multidisciplinary tele-rehabilitation in the assessment and rehabilitation of COVID-19 survivors. International Journal of Environmental Research and Public Health. 2020;**17**:4890. DOI: 10.3390/ijerph17134890

[87] Zhang MW, Ho RC. Moodle: The cost effective solution for internet cognitive behavioral therapy (I-CBT) interventions. Technology and Health Care. 2017;**25**:163-165. DOI: 10.3233/THC-161261

[88] Ho CS, Chee CY, Ho RC. Mental health strategies to combat the psychological impact of coronavirus disease 2019 (COVID-19) beyond paranoia and panic. Annals of the Academy of Medicine, Singapore. 2020;**49**:155-160

[89] Vugts MAP, Joosen MCW, van der Geer JE, Zedlitz AMEE, Vrijhoef HJM. The effectiveness of various computer-based interventions for patients with chronic pain or functional somatic syndromes: A systematic review and meta-analysis. PLoS One. 2018;**13**:e0196467. DOI: 10.1371/journal.pone.0196467

[90] Eccleston C, Fisher E, Craig L, Duggan GB, Rosser BA, Keogh E.

Psychological therapies (Internet-delivered) for the management of chronic pain in adults. Cochrane Database of Systematic Reviews. 2014;**2014**:CD010152. DOI: 10.1002/14651858.CD010152.pub2

[91] Andersson G, Cuijpers P, Carlbring P, Riper H, Hedman E. Guided internet-based vs. face-to-face cognitive behavior therapy for psychiatric and somatic disorders: A systematic review and meta-analysis. World Psychiatry. 2014;**13**:288-295. DOI: 10.1002/wps.20151

[92] Carnes D, Homer KE, Miles CL, Pincus T, Underwood M, Rahman A, et al. Effective delivery styles and content for self-management interventions for chronic musculoskeletal pain: A systematic literature review. Clinical Journal of Pain. 2012;**28**:344-354. DOI: 10.1097/AJP.0b013e31822ed2f3

[93] Brigo E, Rintala A, Kossi O, Verwaest F, Vanhoof O, Feys P, et al. Using telehealth to guarantee the continuity of rehabilitation during the COVID-19 pandemic: A systematic review. International Journal of Environmental Research and Public Health. 2022;**19**:10325. DOI: 10.3390/ijerph191610325

[94] Vadivel R, Shoib S, El Halabi S, El Hayek S, Essam L, Gashi Bytyçi D, et al. Mental health in the post-COVID-19 era: Challenges and the way forward. General Psychiatry. 2021;**34**:e100424. DOI: 10.1136/gpsych-2020-100424

[95] Barach P, Fisher SD, Adams MJ, Burstein GR, Brophy PD, Kuo DZ, et al. Disruption of healthcare: Will the COVID pandemic worsen non-COVID outcomes and disease outbreaks? Progress in Pediatric Cardiology. 2020;**59**:101254. DOI: 10.1016/j.ppedcard.2020.101254

[96] Vindegaard N, Benros ME. COVID-19 pandemic and mental health consequences: Systematic review of the current evidence. Brain, Behavior, and Immunity. 2020;**89**:531-542. DOI: 10.1016/j.bbi.2020.05.048

Chapter 5

Coronavirus 19 (COVID-19) and Syndrome of Inappropriate Anti-Diuretic Hormone Secretion (SIADH): A Review of Literature

Mohammed Somaili

Abstract

The current coronavirus disease (COVID-19) pandemic, caused by the severe acute respiratory distress syndrome coronavirus 2 (SARS-CoV-2) is a serious public health concern worldwide. Over time, it became more evident that COVID-19 can affect multiple endocrine organs and hormonal substances, eventually negatively affecting patients with COVID-19 infection. The mechanism underlying hyponatremia in patients with COVID-19 is not fully understood but many postulated hypotheses have been tested. The exact mechanism of hyponatremia following COVID-19 infection also has yet to be established. The management options in those patients need to be taken carefully and to be directed to the primary disease. In this chapter, we summarize the association of syndrome of inappropriate anti-diuretic hormone secretion (SIADH)-induced hyponatremia with COVID-19 infection.

Keywords: COVID-19, SIADH, hyponatremia, extrapulmonary organs, angiotensin-converting enzyme 2 (ACE2)

1. Introduction

Coronavirus disease (COVID-19) pandemic is caused by the severe acute respiratory distress syndrome coronavirus 2 (SARS-CoV-2) [1, 2]. It represents a global health burden and associated with increased morbidity and mortality. COVID-19 has a diverse and variable spectrum of clinical presentations. The clinical presentations range from mild disease with just upper respiratory tract symptoms to a severe form of the disease including pneumonia and may be multiple organ failure [3].

It became evident that COVID-19 can also affect the extrapulmonary organs, this includes vascular, cardiac, renal and neurological systems [4–7]. Over time, it became more evident that COVID-19 can affect multiple endocrine organs and hormonal substances, leading to negative patients' outcomes. The COVID-19 endocrine manifestations can be found more frequently in those patients with pituitary diseases, diabetes mellitus, obesity and vitamin D deficiency [8].

IntechOpen

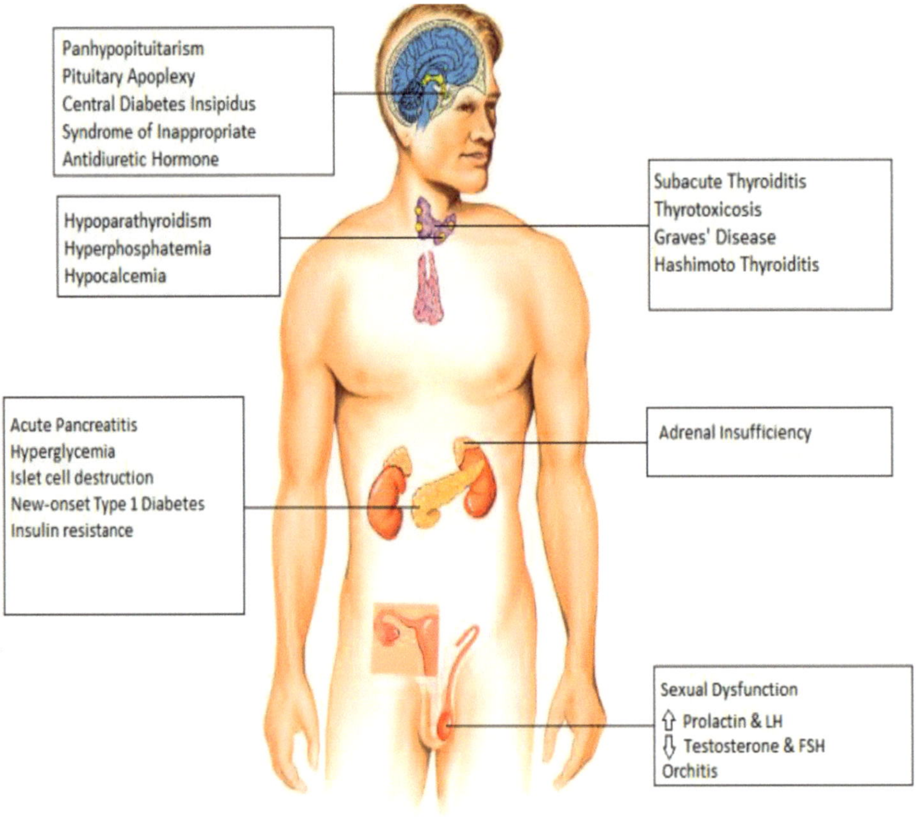

Figure 1.
Endocrine COVID-19 manifestations [11].

Angiotensin-converting enzyme 2 (ACE2) receptors have been identified as a target for the entry SARS-CoV-2 into the cells. The systemic involvement in COVID-19 is due to the almost abundant expression of the angiotensin-converting enzyme 2 (ACE2) receptors, with resulting damage at many organ and tissue levels besides the lung [9, 10]. From the endocrine glands respective, these receptors have been found in the hypothalamus, thyroid, pancreatic, gonads, pituitary gland cells on biopsies from those patients who died from COVID-19, explaining the endocrine involvement after contracting the infection, **Figure 1** [11].

From the initial period of the pandemic, multiple factors have been linked to a higher risk for mortality from COVID-19, including male gender, old age, obesity, DM, hypertension (HTN), cancer, chronic obstructive pulmonary disease, immunocompromised patients and patients with cardiovascular diseases [12].

2. Syndrome of inappropriate secretion of antidiuretic hormone (SIADH)

The syndrome of inappropriate secretion of antidiuretic hormone (SIADH) is characterized by impaired water excretion secondary to the inability to inhibit antidiuretic hormone (ADH) secretion for multiple reasons, which lead eventually to different clinical presentations including hyponatremia [13, 14].

SIADH-induced hyponatremia in COVID-19 patients is not fully understood. One of the speculated hypotheses is related to burst release of inflammatory cytokines, including interleukin IL-1 and IL-6. IL-6 triggers hypothalamic arginine vasopressin production with consequent hyponatremia [15, 16].

SIADH should be considered in the differential diagnosis of any patient presented with hyponatremia (serum sodium levels <135 mmol/L) particularly when it associated with plasma hypo-osmolality, diluted urine and high urinary sodium (>40 mEq/L). Notably and unlike other causes of euvolemic hyponatremia like adrenal insufficiency, in SIADH, the serum potassium level is normal, no acid-base disturbance is observed and the serum uric acid level is frequently low [17].

3. COVID-19 and SIADH-induced hyponatremia

The exact mechanism of hyponatremia following COVID-19 infection has yet to be well established. However, the animal models speculated that it could be due to an imbalance in the intravascular fluid volume and extracellular fluid osmolality. Low volume intravascularly would activate the osmoreceptor and increase the ADH secretion [15].

Stresses, whether physical or non-physical, caused by infection for an instance, as in COVID-19, trigger the hypothalamus-pituitary axis, which leads to ADH secretion. In addition, lung involvement due to COVID-19 resulted in ventilation-perfusion mismatch leading to hypoxic pulmonary vasoconstriction, eventually filling the left atrium. The inability of the left atrium to stretch appropriately and as a consequent of this filling, the ADH will be released, **Figure 2** [18].

Several studies have reported that the association of pneumonia with SIADH; however, few case reports have discussed SIADH secondary to COVID-19 pneumonia [19, 20].

One of observed initial COVID-19 clinical manifestation was SIADH. The potential mechanism was attributed to sepsis and cytokine storm associated with it (excessive IL-6 release), which in turn leads to hypothalamic–pituitary axis activation and subsequent uncontrolled release of anti-diuretic hormone (ADH) [15, 16].

Rizki et al. recently had published a systematic review and meta-analysis to assess the prognostic value of hyponatremia in COVID-19 patients. They found that SIADH-induced hyponatremia was associated with longer intensive care unit (ICU) stay and high mortality rate [21]. This could be explained by water retention induced by high levels of the ADH. Intravascular fluid retention can lead to extravasation due to increased capillary permeability in patients with COVID-19 sepsis which may subsequently increase the requirements of ventilator settings and ICU stay [15, 16, 21–23].

Critical levels of hyponatremia can lead to serious neurological manifestations including seizures, loss of consciousness and even death due to cerebral edema and brain stem compression. On the other hand, rapid correction of hyponatremia can lead to devastating neurological insult such as the osmotic demyelination syndrome [7, 24]. Therefore, proper management of covid-19 infection may result in decreased cytokine storms and eventually decreased ADH secretion [25, 26]. The decision of fluid administration in patients with sepsis as an attempt to improve the hydration and circulation status needs to be taken very carefully. Desalination is a phenomenon in which administration of normal saline in patients with SIADH-induced hyponatremia leads to worsening of hyponatremia. The hypothesized mechanism of this phenomenon is related to the excretion of some of the administered fluids in

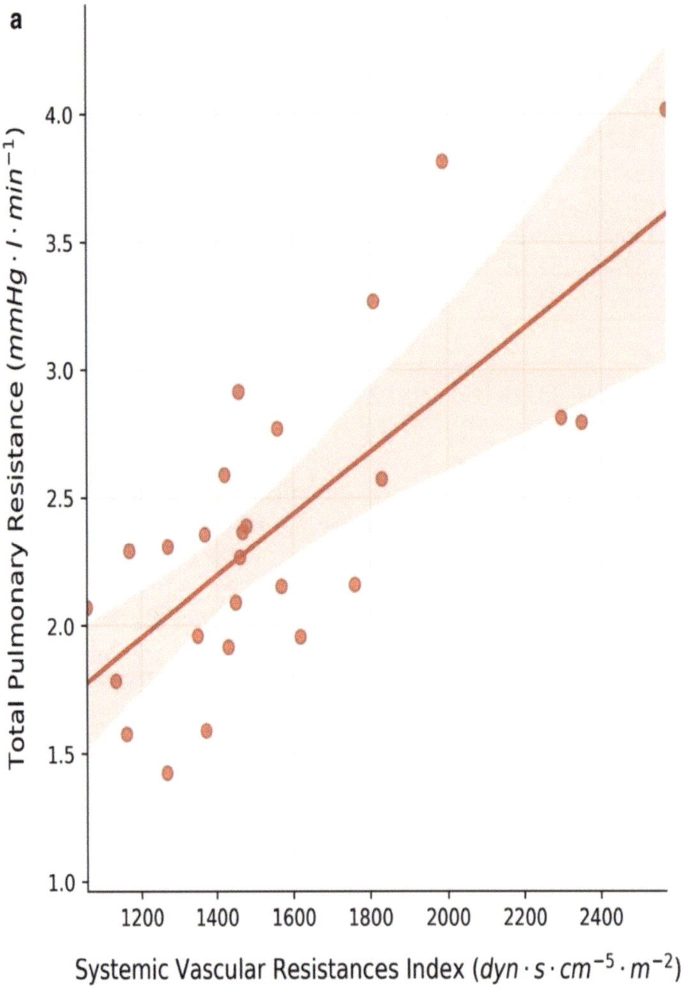

Figure 2.
Hemodynamic changes in early COVID-19 infection [18].

the hyperosmolar urine leaving the remaining in the circulation which leads to more hypotonic plasma and therefore worsening of pre-existing hyponatremia [24, 27]. Thus, the primary target in treating those patients is to the primary disease i.e. the COVID-19 infection. This will consequently lead to improvement of SIADH-induced hyponatremia and improved patients' outcomes.

4. Conclusion

COVID-19 is associated with the development of SIADH; therefore, this condition should be considered in the differential diagnosis in patients with hyponatremia. Administration of IVF warrants cautious decision-making in these settings to avoid worsening of hyponatremia.

Author details

Mohammed Somaili
Department of Medicine, Jazan University, Jizan, Saudi Arabia

*Address all correspondence to: misomaili@jazanu.edu.sa

IntechOpen

© 2023 The Author(s). Licensee IntechOpen. This chapter is distributed under the terms of the Creative Commons Attribution License (http://creativecommons.org/licenses/by/3.0), which permits unrestricted use, distribution, and reproduction in any medium, provided the original work is properly cited.

References

[1] Acter T, Uddin N, Das J, Akhter A, Choudhury TR, Kim S. Evolution of severe acute respiratory syndrome coronavirus 2 (SARS-CoV-2) as coronavirus disease 2019 (COVID-19) pandemic: A global health emergency. Science of the Total Environment. 2020;**730**:138996

[2] Rajgor DD, Lee MH, Archuleta S, Bagdasarian N, Quek SC. The many estimates of the COVID-19 case fatality rate. The Lancet Infectious Diseases. 2020;**20**(7):776-7

[3] Miller R, Englund K. Clinical presentation and course of COVID-19. Cleveland Clinic Journal of Medicine. 2020;**87**(7):384-388

[4] Behzad S, Aghaghazvini L, Radmard AR, Gholamrezanezhad A. Extrapulmonary manifestations of COVID-19: Radiologic and clinical overview. Clinical Imaging. 2020;**66**:35-41

[5] Bansal M. Cardiovascular disease and COVID-19. Diabetes and Metabolic Syndrome: Clinical Research & Reviews. 2020;**14**(3):247-250

[6] Kunutsor SK, Laukkanen JA. Renal complications in COVID-19: A systematic review and meta-analysis. Annals of Medicine. 2020;**52**(7):345-353

[7] Ahmad I, Rathore FA. Neurological manifestations and complications of COVID-19: A literature review. Journal of Clinical Neuroscience. 2020;**77**:8-12

[8] Kazakou P, Paschou SA, Psaltopoulou T, Gavriatopoulou M, Korompoki E, Stefanaki K, et al. Early and late endocrine complications of COVID-19. Endocrine Connections. 2021;**10**(9):R229-R239

[9] Li W, Moore MJ, Vasilieva N, Sui J, Wong SK, Berne MA, et al. Angiotensin-converting enzyme 2 is a functional receptor for the SARS coronavirus. Nature. 2003;**426**(6965):450-454

[10] Ishiyama Y, Gallagher PE, Averill DB, Tallant EA, Brosnihan KB, Ferrario CM. Upregulation of angiotensin-converting enzyme 2 after myocardial infarction by blockade of angiotensin II receptors. Hypertension. 2004;**43**(5):970-976

[11] Mirza SA, Sheikh AAE, Barbera M, Ijaz Z, Javaid MA, Shekhar R, et al. COVID-19 and the endocrine system: A review of the current information and misinformation. Infectious Disease Reports. 2022;**14**(2):184-197

[12] Biswas M, Rahaman S, Biswas TK, Haque Z, Ibrahim B. Association of sex, age, and comorbidities with mortality in COVID-19 patients: A systematic review and meta-analysis. Intervirology. 2021;**64**(1):36-47

[13] Bartter FC, Schwartz WB. The syndrome of inappropriate secretion of antidiuretic hormone. The American Journal of Medicine. 1967;**42**(5):790-806

[14] Vantyghem MC, Balavoine AS, Wémeau JL, Douillard C. Hyponatremia and antidiuresis syndrome. Annales d'Endocrinologie. 2011;**72**(6):500-512

[15] de la José Carlos Flor M, Francisco Valga A, Alexander M, del Miguel Rodeles P. Hyponatremia in COVID-19 infection-possible causal factors and management. Journal of Clinical Nephrology and Renal Care. 2020;**1**:53-56

[16] Gheorghe G, Ilie M, Bungau S, Stoian AMP, Bacalbasa N, Diaconu CC. Is there a relationship between COVID-19

and hyponatremia? Medicina (Mex). 2021;**57**(1):55

[17] Siragy HM. Hyponatremia, fluid-electrolyte disorders, and the syndrome of inappropriate antidiuretic hormone secretion: Diagnosis and treatment options. Endocrine Practice. 2006;**12**(4):446-457

[18] Busana M, Schiavone M, Lanfranchi A, Battista Forleo G, Ceriani E, Beatrice Cogliati C, et al. Non-invasive hemodynamic profile of early COVID-19 infection. Physiological Reports. 2020;**8**:e14628

[19] Somaili M, Abu-aishah H, Haidar W, Hamzi S, Khubrany S. Kidney transplant recipient with syndrome of inappropriate antidiuretic hormone secretion (SIADH) secondary to COVID-19 pneumonia: A case report. Transplantation Proceedings. 2022;**54**(6):1539-1542

[20] Habib MB, Sardar S, Sajid J. Acute symptomatic hyponatremia in setting of SIADH as an isolated presentation of COVID-19. IDCases. 2020;**21**:e00859

[21] Akbar MR, Pranata R, Wibowo A, Irvan STA, Martha JW. The prognostic value of hyponatremia for predicting poor outcome in patients with COVID-19: A systematic review and meta-analysis. Frontiers in Medicine. 2021;**8**:666949

[22] Bermejo-Martin JF, Martín-Fernandez M, López-Mestanza C, Duque P, Almansa R. Shared features of endothelial dysfunction between sepsis and its preceding risk factors (aging and chronic disease). Journal of Clinical Medicine. 2018;**7**(11):400

[23] Meade MO, Cook DJ, Guyatt GH, Slutsky AS, Arabi YM, Cooper DJ, et al. Ventilation strategy using low tidal volumes, recruitment maneuvers, and high positive end-expiratory pressure for acute lung injury and acute respiratory distress syndrome: A randomized controlled trial. Journal of the American Medical Association. 2008;**299**(6):637

[24] King JD, Rosner MH. Osmotic demyelination syndrome. The American Journal of the Medical Sciences. 2010;**339**(6):561-567

[25] Hajjar LA, Leme AC, Rizk SI, Biselli B, Gomes BR, Bittar CS, et al. Intensive care management of patients with COVID-19: A practical approach. Annals of Intensive Care. 2021;**11**(1):36

[26] Poston JT, Patel BK, Davis AM. Management of Critically ill adults with COVID-19. JAMA. 2020;**323**(18):1839-1841

[27] Sterns RH, Hix JK, Silver SM. Management of Hyponatremia in the ICU. Chest. 2013;**144**(2):672-679

Chapter 6

Impact of COVID-19 on Mental Health of Oncology Healthcare Workers and Interdisciplinary Collaboration

Maja Kuzmanovic, Agnieszka Bienert and Klaus Meier

Abstract

The 2019 coronavirus pandemic has caused serious health crises around the world such as psychological reactions of health workers. The way we work (stress, anxiety) and the activities assigned to pharmacists, such as vaccination, have changed. In addition to these problems, numerous ethical questions and moral doubts are increasingly emerging are inevitable during the treatment and care of patients in this extremely difficult situation. Work in the oncology department is stressful even when there is no epidemic/pandemic. Constant changes in hospital protocols, reorganization of work, influx of patients, work in intensive conditions and other new challenges of adaptation to the new situation affect both the physical and mental health of healthcare workers. Together with physicians and nurses, pharmacists were one of the professional categories most exposed to the risk of SARS- CoV-2 infection since the pandemic onset. Together with this crisis, pharmaceutical care entered a new phase demonstrating the ability of pharmacists to be competent and accessible providers of public health. Preserving the mental health of healthcare workers are very important so that they can perform their work with quality and conscientiousness. Health care corporations should consider providing coverage for mental health treatment for employees who experience COVID-19 traumas.

Keywords: COVID-19, healthcare workers, interdisciplinary collaboration, mental health, oncology

1. Introduction

The coronavirus first appeared in the world at the end of 2019 in Wuhan, China. Very fast the virus spread beyond the borders of China, a global pandemic prevailed. Soon scientists identified a new strain of the virus that the World Health Organization named severe acute respiratory syndrome coronavirus 2 or SARS-CoV-2 for short. The disease has become better known as COVID-19 and has become part of the everyday life of people around the world. The virus continues to spread at a high speed and affects an increasing number of patients, and the death rate is increasing every day.

COVID-19 is currently the biggest global and health problem that countries are trying to deal with by introducing numerous epidemiological measures and maintaining social distance [1]. Although the appearance of the virus itself has taught us a lot so far, there are still many uncertainties regarding this virus, its origin, development, and spread of the disease, and they are being considered every day and applying new methods in the treatment. COVID-19 has changed the world and affected it in many aspects, and it left a big mark on the healthcare system. Increasing volume of work, increased number of seriously ill patients and dying patients, sick nurses, and thus a lack of staff to work are just some in a series of numerous problems that appeared or became even more pronounced during these pandemics. In addition to these problems, numerous ethical questions and moral doubts are increasingly emerging and are inevitable during the treatment and care of patients in this extremely difficult situation. COVID-19 put "on the second plan" the treatment of all other diseases in order to prevent the spread of the virus and the risk from the disease of immunocompromised and palliative patients. However, although the primary goal of this is to protect patients from even greater complications, it often has the opposite effect because certain therapies and examinations are delayed and the patient is not able to receive the appropriate one healthcare and protection. Infection with the coronavirus can cause numerous symptoms and signs of the disease. Considering the severity of the disease, symptoms can be divided into mild, medium, and severe. They are mostly connected with the respiratory tract, but numerous nonspecific symptoms of the disease may also be present; the diagnosis of the disease can often be difficult or the disease is not recognized in time. Respiratory symptoms of the disease are often very similar to a cold or the flu, so it is very important to distinguish whether it is a viral infection or flu, because the method of treatment and further procedure with the patient depends on it. Some of the most common symptoms of most patients are dry cough, elevated body temperature, rhinorrhea, headache, general weakness, and muscle pain [2]. Somewhat rarer and nonspecific symptoms of the disease can be nausea, loss of appetite, vomiting, and diarrhea. In very few cases, skin changes in the form of a small red dotted rash were also observed. Also, a symptom which appears very often and can be one of the first signs of the coronavirus is the loss of the sense of taste and smell (anosmia), which can be absent for several weeks after healing. Severe symptoms of the disease include pressure and pain in the chest, dyspnea, difficulty breathing, and feeling of suffocation. Patients with these symptoms should be hospitalized immediately for the treatment. Based on previous analyses, the average incubation is 5.1 days, and an infected person develops symptoms within 11.5 days of infections [3]. Lifestyle habits can play a big role in recovery, which can positively or negatively affect the repair, depending on the life habits of the person. Recovery is slowed down if the person is undisciplined and does not follow health instructions. For example, continued smoking, bad eating habits, too much fatigue from heavy physical activities instead of resting, not taking prescribed therapy on time, refusing therapy and the like, all that may slow down or prevent recovery. There are numerous health conditions that require special attention because the health condition of these persons is in itself impaired. Therefore, it is necessary to look at all the risks that may come into consideration. Extremely sensitive groups of patients, regardless of age, are people who have a transplanted organ, people who suffer from some malignant disease, people who have a certain autoimmune disease, people with severe lung diseases such as asthma and cystic fibrosis, people suffering from extremely rare diseases that are prone to severe infections such as combined immunodeficiency, people using high doses of immunosuppressants' medicines, pregnant women with severe heart disease, and people with any heart disease. All of these diseases and conditions should be kept in mind, and first of all protective measures should be taken to prevent the occurrence of the disease. It is the best method of preventing any complications and unwanted deaths. There are many aspects of staying in the workplace with increased risk of infection which may affect both mental health and well-being. COVID-19 is a contagious disease, and healthcare workers must deal with potentially harmful problems like prolonged fear of being infected and spreading the disease to the family members, insufficient supplies in personal protective equipment, inconvenience of wearing them, extended working hours, sudden changes in a work schedule, additional tasks, excess work, pressure as well as prejudice and social fears. In response, workers may develop a range of behavioral (e.g., effects on performance), physical (e.g., headache, gastric disorders, etc.), and psychological (e.g., mood swings, decreased motivation, depressed thoughts, and isolation) reactions [4]. Concerns are now being raised about the mental health, psychological adjustment, and recovery of health professionals treating and caring for patients with COVID-19. This pandemic poses a major challenge to social, economic, and, above all, the psychological resources of the population. Undoubtedly, healthcare workers are the most exposed category. Supporting the mental health of healthcare workers is a critical part of the public health response.

2. Consequences of mental health in oncology health workers

Cancer is a serious disease, probably the most serious of all, and treatment is very important. The information we constantly receive about COVID-19 can be disturbing. People who have overcome cancer or are still struggling with a malignant disease, as well as their loved ones, can be very worried, considering that this disease and its therapy can reduce the body's ability to fight the coronavirus infection. Maintaining physical distance, frequent and thorough hand washing, avoiding gathering in groups, disinfecting surfaces, and avoiding touching the face with unwashed hands can be a good strategy for everyone, but strict adherence to these measures is especially important for oncology patients who may be immunocompromised. The term "immunocompromised" refers to individuals whose immune system is considered significantly weaker compared to the immune system of a healthy adult. The primary role of the immune system is to defend the body against infections. "Immunocompromised" people are at a higher risk of being infected with an infectious disease, such as the viral infection of COVID-19. There are many reasons why the immune system can be weakened, among others: if a person suffers from cancer, diabetes, heart disease, if the person is elderly or if he is a smoker. Oncology patients have a significantly higher risk of their immune system becoming "compromised" or weakened. It mostly depends on the type of cancer, the type of oncology therapy they receive, their age, and other existing diseases. The risk is greatest at the time of active oncological treatment, i.e. during the period when the patient receives chemotherapy. There is no exact test that can determine whether someone is "immunocompromised" or not, but based on blood findings such as a reduced number of white blood cells or a reduced number of antibodies (immunoglobulins), it can be concluded that the immune system is significantly weakened [5]. Stress at work, i.e. critical incidents with which oncologists meet, can cause symptoms post-traumatic stress, anxiety, depression, and syndrome combustion. Factors that most often cause stress in working with oncology patients are the following: the severity of the diagnosed disease, the increase in the patient's expectations, unsatisfactory care for the patient, the inability of the doctor to control the outcome of the results of his own work and care for the patient, problems related to the patient's family, lack of staff and technology in order to provide the patient with appropriate treatment, too much responsibility of the doctor, communication problems within the team that cares for the patient, too much workload, administrative problems mechanism, working conditions, low salaries, inadequate social support, the status of young newly employed doctors, the end of a doctor's career, lack of opportunities for promotion, decline, and reducing the feeling of gratitude of patients and superiors [6]. Work in the oncology department is stressful even when there is no epidemic/pandemic. Because in the most active phase of life, work takes away most of the time it is to be expected that the work environment will become a source of great stress and loads. Accumulation of stress is the most common cause of mental difficulties, while anxiety is the most common condition with which nurses and technicians in oncology, but also in nursing in general, they meet almost every day. In nursing practice, there is often an excessive workload, but too little load can also be a cause of stress. Too little load is the result of repetitive, routine, and insufficiently stimulating work tasks. Quantitative work overload implies too many tasks in a given period of time, while qualitative indicates a lack of knowledge and experience in performing certain tasks. Both types of work overload and lack of time to perform tasks are significant risk factors in the development of anxiety and depression. Overtime, shift work and on-call combined with night work affect the bio-psychophysical rhythm of a person's functioning. Accompanying complaints appear in the form of chronic fatigue, decreased immunity, gastrointestinal disorders, headaches, and others. Work with antineoplastic therapy is by its nature stressful due to its complexity, and potential complications can cause fear of making a mistake and at the same time additionally endanger a person's life which is going through its own stressful, and in some cases, traumatic experience. On the other hand, the work of cytostatics potentially endangers the health of the person who prepares and applies the therapy and comes into contact with bodily secretions of a person undergoing active treatment. The demandingness of this part of healthcare can impose a sense of personal responsibility for the patient's health and life. In addition to the harmfulness of the therapy, the potential risk and danger for the healthcare workers are represented by the patients with serious mental disorders as a result of primary mental illness and/or secondary in relation to the diagnosis of a malignant disease or the use of certain drugs. In addition to the harmfulness of the therapy, the potential risk and danger for the healthcare workers are represented by the patients with serious mental disorders as a result of primary mental illness and/or secondary in relation to the diagnosis of a malignant disease or the use of certain drugs. Epidemics and pandemics uniquely threaten health, because effective treatment or medicine is often not available. Unlike other types of emergencies, these threats to health can take a long time, with a high degree of uncertainty about progression or disease control. Healthcare workers were involved in the fight during every epidemic/pandemic and risked their lives. In such emergency situations, high-risk situations subject to numerous competing duties, such as duties toward patients, protection from unnecessary risk of injury, duty toward family, colleagues, and society, which can cause great stress and even lead to long-term psychological consequences. Symptoms associated with mental health problems predominantly included expression, anxiety, or stress. This can lead to additional cognitive and social problems, as well as long-term problems, including post-traumatic stress disorder (PTSD). These problems can affect the function in the workplace and negatively at work environments can lead to mental health problems. Each person reacts and focuses on stressful situations differently. Some focus on solving the problem, while others deny reality, struggle with change, feel guilty, or withdraw. If stress exceeds human strength and exhausts the ability to cope, it can lead to pathological reactions. Among other things, stress is responsible for reducing professional satisfaction and well-being of the individual, as well as stagnation in personal development, absence from work, reduction in quality of service, or more errors. The pandemic has a significant emotional impact on patients but also on health workers who are in charge of helping the infected. Their workload is further increased by the high and persistent risk of exposure and death, by separation from their loved ones, which may be forced or due to extended work shifts. Watching of traumatic images of their seriously ill or dying patients in an overloaded environment with chronically low drug supplies, experiencing hopelessness due to large human losses despite all efforts to provide care, management of human bodies, experiencing quarantine, witnessing the death of their colleagues, lack of reinforcements and replacement, fatigue, and burnout are just some of the traumas they have to endure during the course of work. Supporting the mental health of healthcare workers is a critical part of the public health response. Not only did the pandemic change the way and the conditions we work in, bringing with it stress, anxiety, and other psychological problems, but also did it change the tasks and activities assigned to pharmacists. One of the most significant changes the COVID-19 pandemic brought to the pharmacy practice was vaccination. Prior to Covid-19, the vaccination service delivery was available in a limited number of countries; during the worldwide response to the pandemic, it became a routine service delivered by pharmacists (among other healthcare workers) in various settings. Although the approval/authorization of vaccines against SARS-CoV-2 meant having new and effective means of fighting against the virus and at the same time the beginning of the control of the pandemic, it also probably brought up more questions than answers. Would the vaccines be safe? Would they be effective? How will the vaccines be distributed? And stored? Who will prepare them and administer them? Massive administration of the doses all around the globe would provide equally massive amounts of clinically relevant data. Mental health is a prerequisite and fundamental determinant of quality of life. Research on the psychological effects of outbreaks of infectious diseases such as SARS epidemics and H1N1 pandemics on mental health shows consistent patterns of responses by healthcare workers. Staffing challenges include not only increased workloads that create such epidemics and pandemics but also the fear of the possibility of infecting oneself, one's family, and loved ones. Working in a new environment where protocols are often changed, personal protective equipment is applied, with overtime, and most importantly providing caring for the sick in new circumstances causes a great mental burden in healthcare workers. In many cases, the infection spreads rapidly and as it is seen with the COVID-19 infection, difficult decisions had to be made, for example, about who is suitable for intensive treatment and who is not. They understand the gravity of the situation very well, healthcare workers, and less so by the public, which makes it difficult to adapt to the situation for the purpose of adherence to epidemiological measures. Infection control measures and use of personal protective equipment put healthcare workers in aggravating circumstances due to more difficult communication with patients, and staff may feel guilty that such isolated patients "die alone." Many healthcare workers will become infected, with the possibility of developing a severe form of disease that can result in death. Research has shown that health workers who had to go into isolation feel guilty for leaving the "front" and colleagues.

They also fear the possibility of infecting their families, loved ones, and patients. As the profession of a healthcare worker is a profession which has an increased tendency for teamwork, in quarantine health workers suffer from loneliness, boredom, and exhaustion. The COVID-19 pandemic has caused many changes in our lives. Numerous challenges have emerged that need to be addressed, both in professional and private life. Uncertain forecasts, inability to plan and forecast, measures of limited movement, job losses, and financial losses are just some of the stressors. Cancer patients, whose immunity is compromised by therapies, belong to the most at-risk group and are justifiably concerned about their health. They need to be reassured but advised to follow all instructions. In individual counseling, oncology patients should be helped to organize their daily routine, as everyone who is in self-isolation is advised. The only difference is that patients need to continue their treatment, and their outings from the safe home, to be reduced as much as possible, just to go to therapy. All other consultations with physicians should be conducted by telephone or online communications. In addition to patients who are already being treated for cancer, those patients who have just been diagnosed with a malignant disease also feel great fear. They are afraid that treatment will be delayed, and because of that, the treatment outcomes will not be good either. Ultimately, as a risk group, they fear infection more than nonrisk individuals, because the mortality of oncology patients infected with the coronavirus virus is far higher than the mortality in the general population. But cancer mortality is far higher, and they should be encouraged to continue their treatment. People who have some symptoms that may indicate the appearance of malignancy should be advised to go to their family doctor, to check if they can postpone the tests or to do them if the doctor advises. The data of some hospitals that they have fewer registered oncology patients is worrying. This does not mean that the incidence has dropped, but that patients do not go to the doctors for fear of the corona virus.

3. Multidisciplinary approach in the treatment of COVID-19

What seems most important, at the time of a pandemic, is that patients receive all the important information. The source of information must be professional, high quality, and reliable. A quality source of information is reflected in a multidisciplinary team. Multidisciplinary teams and the integration of a clinical/oncology pharmacist are necessary for optimal oncology care. By introducing consultation with a clinical/oncology pharmacist, who focuses on relevant issues, it significantly raises the quality of life, explaining the therapy itself, and emotionally preparing for what follows. Caring for patients during an epidemic/pandemic may impact negatively on the mental health of healthcare workers. The psychological responses of healthcare workers to the pandemic of infectious diseases are complicated. In a short time period, healthcare workers used a large part of their abilities in controlling how to spend their time, where to direct their attention, and how best to use scarce resources. The foundation of best care for cancer patients is without a doubt the well-being of oncology healthcare workers, where burnout has been most extensively studied. Burnout phenomenon and prevention among oncologists were known to be significant even before COVID-19 pandemic; however, it has gained strength since the global influence of coronavirus on healthcare system. The long-term nature and scope of this impact are still unknown. High level of anxiety has been noticed among oncology healthcare workers during the first period of COVID-19 pandemic in the United States and Singapore [7, 8]. Actually, physicians of various specializations suffer from the distress caused by COVID-19. In the study from Wuhan, China, the authors noticed that oncologists and nurses working directly with COVID-19 patients did not deal with such significant burnout like their colleagues who stayed in their familiar/previous settings. According to authors' opinion, the reason of this can be greater feeling of control due to direct involvement and mobilization connected with fighting with COVID-19. Thus, it can be concluded that the impact of COVID-19 on mental health and well-being is complex as well as it differs between regions and specializations [9]. Daily work with seriously ill patients had consequences for all members of the healthcare team. Nurses suffer physical and emotional stress every day, by caring patients and facing numerous ethical and moral challenges that this pandemic has brought with it. Due to insufficient healthcare workers, insufficient resources, and a large number of deaths, nurses are in a conflict of professional values every day. More and more nurses are sick with COVID-19, and some have died as a result of the disease which they received by performing their duty. Due to the large amount of stress and emotional suffering that passes, nurses need great courage, strength, and endurance when working and fighting with this virus, and during that time they are away from their families and loved ones. Patients who suffered from other severe chronic and incurable diseases were put on long waiting lists. The operating theaters were almost completely closed, and only emergency operations were performed. If someone got sick or had an accident, they should be hours in order to be able to come for an examination or to the clinic to dress a wound. Because of the increased costs for procuring protective equipment and all medicines necessary for the treatment of COVID-19, the "budgets" for other medicines and necessities have decreased, so often oncology patients were left without their expensive medicines, which they cannot afford on their own. Chemotherapy and radiation were postponed, so many were in uncertainty as to what would happen to their treatment. An oncology-palliative patient infected with the coronavirus is faced with numerous problems that they still have not managed to solve in the health system. So, it is not uncommon for them to undergo chemotherapy and radiation that are delayed due to lack of space or the impossibility of obtaining medicine. When they come to their own term of therapy, due to epidemiological measures, they mostly remain alone in the room, which is negative. It affects their psychological status because they feel lonely, sad, and rejected, and this can lead to the development of depression. Dissatisfaction was also observed among nurses who work in the oncology and palliative wards because due to the prescribed measures, their income has reduced interaction with the patient, so the psychological part of help and therapeutic communication are almost completely absent. Furthermore, the redistribution of staff due to the need for work in other departments in part of the pandemic leads to some nurses remaining to work with palliative care patients, so the nurses do not have enough time to dedicate themselves equally to each patient because of the scope of work. Similar problems are present in the oncology-palliative patient he visits and who is in home care [10]. Due to the lack of teams on the field and the increased number of palliative care users, the same problems develop as in many inpatients healthcare institutions. In addition to numerous organizational problems, lack of personnel, emotional stress caused by work, increased number of patients, ethical issues, and moral doubts making numerous decisions became another big burden during the implementation of palliative care for patients with COVID-19. Due to the increased volume of work and the number of patients due to the pandemic, stress is pronounced more than ever before. Great mental stress, seeing death every day, and great emotional stress pressure led to the psychological burnout of many healthcare workers. Professional burnout has many negative effects on the body and mental health of the individual, which ultimately affects engagement and efficiency in work.

Psychological burnout can be defined as a continuous affective stress reaction that develops over a long period of time and consists of emotional exhaustion, feelings of inadequacy, success, and depersonalization. The most pronounced dimension of psychological burnout is most often emotional exhaustion. It arises due to intense emotional feelings that appear in interaction with patients and ultimately lead to irritability, fatigue, and decreased enthusiasm at work. Caring for the dying, looking death in the eye every day, dealing with dead bodies, and a large number of healthcare workers had an emotional breakdown. The long-term impact of the pandemic is still not fully known on the mental state of healthcare workers, but dealing with other people's suffering, pain, and death contributes to great psychological burnout. Watching how every day more and more young people were dying from this virus left a hard impression on the emotional consequences for health personnel. Shortness of breath, rapid breathing, coughing fits and coughing up large amounts of secretions caused great anxiety and fear in patients. Many nurses and doctors described how the fear of suffocation was present in all patients' lack of air and death and the impossibility of saying goodbye to the family. Due to major traumas and stressful situations experienced at work, healthcare workers are also at risk of developing PTSD (post-traumatic stress disorder). Faced with daily difficult decisions, they often struggle with feelings of guilt and they wonder if all the decisions were made well and if they could have done something better for such difficult patients. Every day they struggle with difficult decisions such as who to resuscitate and which one put the patient on a ventilator, and the biggest feeling of guilt is caused by the fact that due to the large scope work and lack of staff, many patients die alone and have no one to lend a hand to. Because of that harmonization of professional duties, which include making ethical decisions, has brought great pressure at work, and ethics meetings are very rare or almost nonexistent because for them it is simple, there is no time, or it is currently being neglected due to other important matters. Because of the immense courage and help they provide to the entire community, healthcare workers were often referred to by the public and the media as "heroes in white coats." The uncertainty of when humanity will return to normal has become an additional burden and pressure. An unprecedented rate of sadness and depression has been recorded, which can be devastating in the short and long term and affect individuals and society. This is why it is extremely important to take steps to solving long-term psychological stress, especially for health personnel. Self-care should be encouraged, and the support of family and colleagues is crucial and should always be available. In 2020, the medical academy issued a recommendation for the well-being of healthcare workers during the pandemic, including meeting basic human needs, respecting differences, and respect for human rights. The upheaval in the professional role of healthcare workers in dealing with the COVID-19 infection leads to new challenges and adjustments in the entire healthcare sector. Increased education, training, and preparation of health workers for work in crisis situations is one of the more effective measures to alleviate mental pressure for health workers. Therefore, in crisis situations, it is important to strengthen the enthusiasm, knowledge, and conscientiousness of healthcare workers. A closer monitoring of and active intervention for the mental health of healthcare workers should be continued. According to data from the literature, young health workers have more experienced stress levels and have higher anxiety than the elderly. One of the possible reasons why older workers show less symptoms and difficulties with mental health is that many older workers experienced this in their practice and for this reason developed better coping skills. Women can be assumed to be more emotional, and they have a more empathetic attitude toward patients and their families, which consequently leads to excessive self-responsibility for the life and health of patients [11]. Although in these difficult times, healthcare workers provide their services to the maximum, and they still need help and support from their superiors. Psychological treatment such as cognitive behavior therapy and mindfulness therapy could be helpful. In this specific time period passing under the sign of COVID-19 pandemic, healthcare workers should be provided with psychosocial and mental health support, especially the groups, where the risk is high. It is obvious that healthcare workers are willing to be welcomed, listened to, supported, and protected by their organizations. With the spread of SARS-Cov-2 virus and vaccination, we can clearly distinguish three additional responsibilities of pharmacists: vaccine administration allowance (and mostly preparation), issuing of certificate of vaccination, and prescribing allowance. Also, the pandemic accelerated the process of increasing interdisciplinary approach to the patient care which can be certainly viewed as an advantage. On the other hand, new challenges as well as an increase in the workload affect the mental health of healthcare workers. Pharmacists are the most accessible healthcare workers, and their role in the health sector is very significant. The role of pharmacists in hospital and community pharmacies is multiple: experts in drugs and medicines, healthcare providers and stakeholders, educators, counselors, mentors, managers, leaders, business developers, researchers, etc. [12]. Together with physicians and nurses, pharmacists were one of the professional categories most exposed to the risk of SARS-CoV-2 infection since the pandemic onset. Together with this crisis, pharmaceutical care entered a new phase demonstrating the ability of pharmacists to be competent and accessible providers of public health. The inclusion of pharmacists in multidisciplinary teams, during this pandemic, has been very useful and important. Pharmacists gained new experiences and practices, which will certainly be of great use to them for some new challenges in the future. New situation leads to the rapid development of a multiprofessional approach in everyday work, development of certain narrowly specialized areas of professional and scientific work, and standardization of all procedures in the treatment process. This is exactly the foundation of quality-designed pharmacy, medical, and nursing care. It is essential that the support on mental health is fast, to avoid the severe disorders which can lead to dysfunctions, sufferings, and in the extreme cases, when not recognized and treated early enough cause even death. Due to COVID-19 pandemic, healthcare workers have been separated in many different aspects which are very challenging for the society to comprehend. Healthcare corporations should take into account protection and care for employees who experienceCOVID-19 traumas.

Author details

Maja Kuzmanovic[1*], Agnieszka Bienert[2] and Klaus Meier[3]

1 Hospital Pharmacy, Public Institution Cantonal Hospital Zenica, Zenica, Bosnia and Herzegovina

2 Department of Clinical Pharmacy and Biopharmacy, Poznan University of Medical, Sciences, Poznan, Poland

3 Institute for Applied Healthcare Sciences, Germany

*Address all correspondence to: magistra1985@gmail.com

IntechOpen

© 2023 The Author(s). Licensee IntechOpen. This chapter is distributed under the terms of the Creative Commons Attribution License (http://creativecommons.org/licenses/by/3.0), which permits unrestricted use, distribution, and reproduction in any medium, provided the original work is properly cited.

References

[1] Kisely S, Warren N, McMahon L, Dalais C, Henry I, Siskind D. Occurrence, prevention, and management of the psychological effects of emerging virus outbreaks on healthcare workers: Rapid review and meta-analysis. BMJ. 2020;**369**:m1642

[2] Wu D, Wu T, Liu Q, Yang Z. The SARS-CoV-2 Outbreak: What we know. International Journal of Infectious Diseases. 2020;**94**:44-48

[3] Lauer SA, Grantz KH, Bi Q, Jones FK, Zheng Q, Meredith HR, et al. The incubation period of coronavirus disease 2019 (COVID-19) from publicly reported confirmed cases: Estimation and application. Annals of Internal Medicine (Philadelphia, PA). 2020;**172**(9):577-582

[4] Giorgi G, Lecca LI, Alessio F, Finstad GL, Bondanini G, Lulli LG, et al. COVID-19-related mental health effects in the workplace: A narrative review. International Journal of Environmental Research and Public Health. 2020;**17**(21):7857. DOI: 10.3390/ijerph17217857

[5] Cancer. Net. Common Questions About COVID-19 and Cancers: Answers for Patients and Survivors. 2020. Available at: https://www.cancer.net.blog72020/04/

[6] Wong TW, Yau JK, Kwong RS, Chan CL, Kwong RS, Ho SM, et al. The psychological impact of severe acute respiratory syndrome outbreak on healthcare workers in emergenc departments and how they cope. European Journal of Emergency Medicine. 2005;**12**(1):13-18

[7] Ng KYY, Zhou S, Tan SH, Ishak NBD, Goh ZZS, Chua ZY, et al. Understanding the psychological impact of COVID-19 pandemic on patients with cancer, their caregivers, and health Care Workers in Singapore. JCO Global Oncology. 2020;**6**:1494-1509

[8] Thomaier L, Teoh D, Jewett P, Beckwith H, Parsons H, Yuan J, et al. Emotional health concerns of oncology physicians in the United States: Fallout during the COVID-19 pandemic. PLoS One. 2020;**15**(11):e0242767

[9] Wu Y, Wang J, Luo C, Hu S, Lin X, Anderson A, et al. Comparison of burnout frequency among oncology physicians and nurses working on the frontline and usual wards during the COVID-19 epidemic in Wuhan, China. Journal of of Pain and Symptom Management. 2020;**60**(1):e60-e65

[10] Kates J, Gerolamo A, Pogorzelska-Maziarz M. The impact of COVID-19 on the hospice and palliative care workforce. Public Health Nursing. 2021;**38**(3):459-463

[11] Białek K, Sadowski M. Level of stress and strategies used to cope with stress by physicians working in intensive care units. Anaesthesiology Intensive Therapy. 2019;**51**(5):361-369

[12] Elbeddini A, Prabaharan T, Almasalkhi S, Tran C. Pharmacists and COVID-19. Journal of Pharmaceutical Policy and Practice. 2020;**13**:36

Chapter 7

Post-COVID-19 Condition and Its Presence in Mexico

Efraín Navarro-Olivos, Gilberto Flores-Vargas, Guadalupe Irazú Morales-Reyes, Jéssica Paola Plascencia-Roldán, María de Jesús Gallardo-Luna and Nicolás Padilla-Raygoza

Abstract

In this chapter, we discuss general information about the post-COVID-19 condition, also known as long COVID. Since it is still under research, many questions remain unanswered. Nevertheless, post-acute complications due to infections have been previously reported for other viruses. Among those complications that remain are anosmia, fatigue, cardiovascular, and pulmonary. The evidence so far suggests that these complications decrease with time. The most worrying persistent symptoms due to COVID-19 are related to neurological damage. Most post-COVID-19 complications can be treated in a standard way, but their impact on life quality is unknown. Finally, we present a rough landscape of long COVID-19 in Mexico and Latin America. More studies are needed to study this condition and its impact on public health.

Keywords: long COVID-19, post-acute COVID-19, persistent symptoms, fatigue, brain fog

1. Introduction

In December 2019, an outbreak of pneumonia of unknown origin occurred in the City of Wuhan, China [1]. On January 9th, 2020, the virus behind the infections was identified as a new strain of β-coronavirus [2]. Subsequently, on February 11th, it was named by the World Health Organization (WHO) as severe acute respiratory syndrome coronavirus 2 (SARS-CoV-2), and the associated disease was coronavirus disease 2019 (COVID-19) [2].

According to an interim WHO guidance for the management of patients with suspected COVID-19 [3], early reports from the China Center Disease Control (CCDC) suggested that most people who developed a confirmed case of COVID-19 infection manifested mild symptoms, 14% developed a severe disease that required hospitalization, of which 5% required admission to the intensive care unit; with a higher risk of death those with advanced age and presence of comorbidities [3].

 IntechOpen

Severe disease and death have been observed in patients older than 75 years. The comorbidities associated with a higher risk of death are hypertension, cardiovascular diseases, diabetes, chronic respiratory diseases, and cancer [4].

The COVID-19 symptoms related to neurological disease reported so far are anosmia, dysgeusia, muscle pain, and headache during the early stage of the infection [5]. These symptoms suggest many hypotheses about how the virus reaches the nervous system. Some of them are its potential entry via the olfactory groove or bloodstream [6–9].

In Mexico, the first official case was reported on February 28th, 2020 [10], and by March 11th, 2020, the WHO declared COVID-19 a global pandemic [11]. Up to May 5th, 2020, 3,525,116 confirmed cases were reported globally, having a case fatality rate of 3.4% [2].

In Mexico, up to January 26th, 2022, the national cumulative incidence rate was 36.00 cases per 1000 inhabitants. Meanwhile, the number of cases was 13,682,501. The mortality rate per 1000 inhabitants in age groups older than 60 was 12.04 [12].

According to Wang et al. [13], the estimated excess mortality in 2020–2021 was 18.2 million people. Mexico has not been the exception since, according to the same study, it is among the countries with the highest excess mortality induced by COVID-19, accounting for 798,000. According to Halabe-Cherem et al. [14], the impact of COVID-19 on health extends beyond disease and mortality rates, affecting the management of chronic conditions, preventive care, and vaccination programs. Moreover, many patients experience physical and mental sequelae that persist for months after recovery from the virus. This persistence of symptoms is known as "prolonged COVID" or "post-COVID syndrome" [14].

2. Sequels due to COVID-19, post-COVID-19 condition, or long COVID-19

Most patients with COVID-19 recover after acute infection with SARS-CoV-2, but some report persistent complications. Michelin et al. [15] conclude that the studies up to 2021 were quite heterogeneous and mostly from Western European countries, with little representation from low to mid-developed countries.

The definition of this disease has changed throughout the pandemic, emerging with various names, including long-term COVID or post-COVID-19 condition [15].

Syndromes due to post-acute infection have previously been reported [16]. According to the review by Choutka et al. [16], the possible causes of these syndromes are remnants or reservoirs of the pathogen that caused the primary infection, autoimmune response, dysbiosis or reactivation, and tissue damage.

In the case of COVID-19, the active SARS-CoV-2 virus has been found even 3 to 6 months after infection [17]. For their part, Wallukat et al. [18] explore the relationship between prolonged COVID and the autoimmune response, finding autoantibodies in most patients who developed long COVID-19. Regarding the last two possible causes of long COVID, gastrointestinal affectations have been reported, in addition to the damage to lung tissues [3].

Prolonged COVID-19 can generate limitations in the daily activities of patients. The situations where a person with long COVID-19 is affected in their daily activities are diverse, for example:

Those with lung damage will have shortness of breath, fatigue, and these effects are mainly related to a limitation in respiratory function [19]. Those presenting with symptoms such as intestinal pain and nausea that have persisted for months are associated with limited gastrointestinal function [19].

People who experience memory problems or "brain fog" suffer from issues related to concentration or thinking [19].

The long-term sequelae generated by COVID-19 are unknown. However, repercussions have been reported worldwide at various systemic levels. These include pulmonary, cardiovascular, neurological, and even mental health. Although these conditions are not lethal, they damage the quality of life. In the case of the Mexican population, these sequelae are associated with the comorbidities that occur most frequently in this population. Long-term complications secondary to COVID-19 could be expected later [20].

The following sections report the most common complications reported in the literature.

2.1 Pulmonary complications

Torres-Cuevas et al. [20] report studies suggesting that approximately 40% of the population infected by SARS-CoV-2 and Middle East Respiratory Syndrome (MERS) presented radiological changes and data suggestive of pulmonary fibrosis, which were associated with respiratory alteration, even 15 years after the infection. The same authors mention the following risk factors:

- Age
- Disease severity
- Stay in intensive care
- Mechanic ventilation
- Smoking and alcoholism
- These factors are expected to play a likewise role in the long COVID-19.

Torres-Cuevas et al. [20] reported that as many as one-third of COVID-19 patients exhibit signs of pulmonary fibrosis and lung function abnormalities 3 months after COVID-19. Pulmonary fibrosis is relevant because it is associated with higher morbidity and mortality. It may also be considered the most significant health sequel of the pandemic since it requires the implementation of pulmonary rehabilitation techniques [20].

Similarly, it has been identified that respiratory symptoms due to COVID-19 can persist even 110 days after the acute picture, the most frequent being chest pain, anosmia, cough, and dyspnea [20].

2.2 Cardiovascular complications

Viruses can cause pericarditis due to systemic inflammation generated in severe cases [21] due to cytotoxic mechanisms. In addition, SARS-CoV-2 infection induces an excessive inflammatory response. This inflammation is responsible for pericardial effusions or cardiac tamponade [20, 22].

Elevated Angiotensin-Converting Enzyme 2 (ACE-2) presence in the cardiovascular system allows direct viral invasion. Then, the immune response and cytokines cause inflammation of the heart muscle, interfering with the conduction system and heart pumping capacity, leading to arrhythmias and cardiac arrest [23].

Infectious processes of viral origin are associated with cardiovascular complications, one of the chief causes of mortality. The effect can persist for up to 10 years after the acute infectious process [20].

Months after the acute phase of SARS-CoV-2 infection, regardless of severity, up to 60% of cases present myocarditis and 71% high-sensitivity troponin T elevation. It is due to a significant decrease in left ventricular ejection fraction [20].

Thrombotic events are considered one of the leading causes of death in patients with COVID-19. Various mechanisms generate a procoagulant state due to an unregulated release of proinflammatory cytokines, resulting in endothelial damage and dysfunction, as an increase in promoters of platelet aggregation and fibrin formation [20].

Different factors favor the presentation of these complications in patients after COVID-19, so an increase in the incidence of this group of diseases in the Mexican population can be expected [20].

2.3 Neurological symptoms and complications

Among the most frequent symptoms are anosmia, headache, myalgias, and mental fog [20].

Neurological alterations are of great relevance since they may significantly affect the quality of life of those who survived COVID-19 [20].

Different viral infections, including coronavirus infections, can manifest with neurosensory alterations, demyelinating diseases, or cerebral vascular events in surviving patients after recovering. After SARS-CoV-2 infection, neuropsychiatric alterations that persisted up to 4 years after recovery were identified [24].

Since the discovery of SARS-CoV-2, various hypotheses have emerged about the mechanism of development of this complication, including its neuroinvasive potential through the olfactory groove or invasion of the nervous system through the bloodstream [24].

Flores-Silva et al. [1] mention that up to 52% of patients may persist with fatigue 10 weeks after the onset of the disease, independent of the severity. This symptom is considered the most frequent in the long term [24].

After the acute phase, about 5–10% of patients persist with anosmia at 4 weeks, with the probability of developing parosmia. In 20–30% of patients, headache is present for 6 weeks, and in 10–20% for up to 9 months. Myalgias are observed during the acute phase, and some patients may present occasional osteoarticular and muscular pain [20].

Other complications from COVID-19 are cerebral vascular events, especially of the ischemic type, which, compared to patients without COVID-19, are usually more severe and have a worse prognosis. The sequelae can hinder the rehabilitation process and even permanently disable the survivors, making it difficult to reintegrate into working and social life. After the acute symptoms of COVID-19, 30% of patients present memory loss, difficulty concentrating, or insomnia. Other reported symptoms are vertigo, headache, and brain fog—discovered as a cognitive alteration, which combines a state of confusion and disorientation [20].

The factors associated with the development of new in-hospital neurological events seem to be related to the severity of the disease, both in respiratory parameters (PaO_2/FiO_2 ratio, Acute Respiratory Distress Syndrome (ARDS) severity, and chest CT findings) and inflammatory markers (C-reactive protein, D-dimer, and neutrophil/lymphocyte ratio) [24].

Flores-Silva et al. [1], by including non-specific neurological manifestations—such as headache, anosmia, dysgeusia, and myalgia—found a frequency of 69.3%, slightly higher than the reported overall frequency of 56.4% [24].

Neurological manifestations, as previously mentioned, have a variable spectrum of presentation, from headache and alterations in taste and smell to ischemic and hemorrhagic cerebrovascular disease [25].

In Mexico, a study carried out at the Specialty Hospital of the Siglo XXI National Medical Center in hospitalized patients with severe COVID-19 identified neurological manifestations in 78 patients (36.4%) out of 214. The most frequent were from the central nervous system: headache, encephalopathy, and cerebrovascular disease (24.8%). The second most were from the peripheral nervous system: anosmia, dysgeusia, and myopathies (8.9%) [25].

Albarran-Sánchez et al. [6] report an incidence of alterations in the sense of smell ranging from 4.9 to 85.6%. The incidence of taste disturbances has been highly variable, ranging from 0.3 to 88.8%, referred to as dysgeusia and ageusia. Finally, headache incidence was from 0.6 to 70.3% [25].

The acute cerebrovascular disease has been associated with COVID-19 with a worse prognosis due to increased mortality. It was also the most frequent neurological manifestation in the study conducted by Albarran-Sanchez et al. [25].

2.4 Anosmia

Anosmia is considered a sequel to COVID-19, caused by damage to the respiratory neuroepithelium. Some studies mention that the damage is driven by the viral invasion of ACE 2 and TMPRSS2 cell receptors—found in the nasal and olfactory epithelium [14].

In the olfactory epithelium, infiltrating leukocytes secrete various proinflammatory cytokines that affect olfactory receptor neurons and the stem cell niche, altering their odorant responses and ability to regenerate [14].

Halabe-Cherem et al. [3] mention that 1 out of 2 patients with COVID-19 will develop anosmia, which affects the quality of life. It influences the ability of people to enjoy smells or detect danger through them [14].

Gutierrez-Bautista et al. [23] observed that 27 of 30 people improved the odor detection threshold 2 months after the onset of the symptoms. Nevertheless, it was not significant in identifying them [23].

2.5 Mental health

In patients with previous SARS-CoV-2 infection, some mental health symptoms prevail up to 2 years later. Identified risk factors are [20]:

- Previous psychiatric illness
- Alcohol
- Unemployment

Regarding COVID-19, an increase in these disorders is expected in the Mexican population since 30.2% of the population over 12 years of age report feelings of depression, 35.5% meet the criteria for excessive alcohol consumption, and a considerable increase in job losses after the pandemic. Within the mental health sequelae secondary to COVID-19, different neuropsychiatric disorders have been identified that can emerge after the acute phase of the disease, as well as an increase in mood-related symptoms, especially in patients with a pre-existing psychiatric illness [20].

A study by Granados-Villalpando et al. [15] which included 203 patients, 96 having prior COVID-19 infection, reported that the most common symptoms of persistent COVID-19 were tiredness, headache, deprivation, and an inconsistent sleep pattern in patients who did not present any previous mental pathology. Meanwhile, in patients who already had some mental pathology before the COVID-19 infection, the symptoms were sleep deprivation, an inconsistent sleep pattern, fatigue, headache, memory problems, brain fog, depression, anxiety, and stress. It shows that the presence of COVID-19 and mental health conditions increases the probability of developing depression, anxiety, or stress [26].

There is a clear relationship between prolonged COVID syndrome and mental disorders [26].

2.6 Obstetric complications

SARS-CoV-2 infection affects pregnant women and fetuses, causing preterm birth, fetal distress, premature rupture of membranes, and cesarean delivery [27].

ACE-2 in the ovary-which plays several functions-could be a potential target of SARS-CoV-2 [27].

Since the architecture of the tissue changes with each renewal of the menstrual cycle, the consequences of SARS-CoV-2 infection, such as menstrual disorders and fertility problems, could be restarted from one to another [23].

2.7 Male reproductive system

Patell et al. [15] analyzed the semen of nine hospitalized patients diagnosed with COVID-19 concluding that 39.1% met the criteria for oligospermia [15].

Expression of ACE-2 and TMPRSS2 in spermatogonia, Leydig cells, and Sertoli cells makes it possible for the virus to invade the testes [23].

The problem leads to cell deterioration, interfering with testosterone release and luteinizing hormone surge, altering sperm production [23].

The released proinflammatory cytokines induce a local inflammatory response that can cause orchitis and systemic inflammation, leading to a persistent fever that ultimately affects sperm morphology, motility, and DNA [28, 29].

Batiha et al. [16] reported normal testosterone levels and decreased testosterone/luteinizing hormone and follicle stimulating hormone/luteinizing hormone ratio without proving causality [28].

3. Treatments

This section presents recommendations for treating post-COVID-19 conditions or complications [30]. In **Table 1**, we summarize the content of this section.

Condition	Treatment	Observed benefit
Fatigue	Rest, supervised exercise, and supplements.	Increase in activity levels.
Neurologic and neurocognitive symptoms.	Neurocognitive rehabilitation.	Improved condition to prior states.
Psychological and emotional problems.	Serotonin reuptake inhibitors or medication according to preexisting conditions.	Improvement of mood and emotions.
Dyspnea and cough.	Breathing exercises and respiratory physiotherapy.	Recovery of normal breathing.
Olfactory-gustatory symptoms.	Supplements and therapy.	Recovery of olfactory-gustatory capacity.

Source: Elaborated by authors from [31, 32].

Table 1.
Conditions and its treatment.

3.1 Fatigue

Fatigue is the appearance of unexplained physical and mental asthenia, which can be persistent or recurrent, leading to a reduction in the patient's activity level [31].

Nowadays, there is no specific treatment, but patients can benefit from the following recommendations and symptom management:

- Rest: it is recommended to have good sleep hygiene (having a regular bedtime and waking hours, avoiding heavy, sugary, stimulant foods, and using computer or mobile screens before sleep). If necessary, consider treatment for sleep problems (melatonin).

- Exercise: it must be controlled and supervised by physiotherapists. It is crucial to carry out personalized and gradual rehabilitation and resume exercising to ease the symptoms associated with post-exercise fatigue or myalgic encephalitis.

- Supplementation: there is a hypothesis that the patient may benefit from the supplementation of coenzyme Q-10, L-carnitine, PQQ, L-Glutamine, or D-Ribose [31].

3.2 Neurologic and neurocognitive symptoms

Cognitive symptoms such as difficulty concentrating, attention problems, and memory failure have been described frequently. These symptoms tend to improve in the long term after performing neurocognitive rehabilitation [31].

Symptomatic treatment should be offered to people with headaches, with the one usually employed for the primary headache they present, depending on the tension or migraine type [31].

There is no pharmacological treatment to speed up smell recovery or to attenuate parosmia. In the case of myalgias, the treatment is symptomatic, where Non-Steroidal Anti-Inflammatory Drugs (NSAIDs) are commonly administered [31].

3.3 Psychological and emotional problems

For those presenting with mild to moderate anxiety and depression, Selective Serotonin Reuptake Inhibitors (SSRIs) should be initiated progressively to maintenance doses with a reassessment every 3–4 weeks [31].

In the case of neuropathic pain or a history of diabetes mellitus, duloxetine would be the antidepressant of choice. If the existing clinical picture includes diarrhea or digestive disorders, the chosen treatment would be paroxetine [31].

3.4 Dyspnea and cough

For mild symptoms of dyspnea that do not require oxygen and do not have a cardiac etiology, they may benefit from breathing exercises and respiratory physiotherapy.

The following is recommended for cough: antitussives such as dextromethorphan or guaifenesin, bronchodilators such as inhaled therapies, bronchodilators, or inhaled glucocorticoids [31].

3.5 Olfactory-gustatory symptoms

If symptoms do not resolve after 2 months, evaluation by an otolaryngologist may be necessary [31].

Treatment consists of olfactory rehabilitation. The use of oral or topical corticosteroid therapy for 15 days, vitamin D, sodium citrate, or theophylline is evaluated, recommending the performance of olfactometry [31].

They could benefit from the stimulation or rehabilitation of smell through occupational therapy or speech therapy [32].

4. Long COVID-19 studies in Mexico and Latin America

In Mexico, a case–control study carried out in the state of Zacatecas with 219 patients found a relative risk of 2 to 33 times higher for developing persistent symptoms such as dyspnea, nausea, and anosmia [20].

An ongoing longitudinal study of neurological syndromes associated with COVID-19 in Mexico City found a high frequency of neurological manifestations during hospitalization in patients with COVID-19, suggesting a higher number of short- and long-term sequelae for these patients [24].

In a follow-up study of patients discharged from a temporary hospital dedicated to COVID-19 in Mexico, the groups of symptoms that presented in more than 30% of the participants 90 days after discharge were neurological, dermatological, and mood disorders. In this study, women presented persistent symptoms more frequently than men, consistent with studies in Wuhan, showing a relationship between the female sex and the symptoms of prolonged COVID-19 [25].

Alvarez-Moreno et al. [33] reported that the most persistent symptoms in Bogotá, Colombia, were headache, fatigue, and insomnia. Likewise, they emphasize that their results are like those reported in other studies. Also, they suggest that there may be an underreporting effect in Latin America that could accentuate social inequalities.

In the study by González-Hermosillo et al. [34], patients who have persistent fatigue for 3 to 6 months were associated with ages between 40 and 50 years.

Patients with fatigue have a high prevalence of other symptoms such as bradypnea, cognitive decline, sleep problems, autonomic dysregulation, and psychological stress. In Mexican studies, the depression and anxiety prevalence among previous COVID-19 patients are up to 15.7% and 22.6%, respectively [34].

The prevalence of symptoms has a progressive decrease with time. A 6-month follow-up study in patients who recovered from the COVID-19 infection showed a reduction in fatigue prevalence—from 53 to 46.9%.

Gonzalez-Hermosillo et al. [34] found that 40.4% of the patients presented persistent symptoms. Of them, 9.1% had a progressive reduction after 4 weeks [34].

5. Conclusions

COVID-19 has a pronounced impact on society, mainly due to its repercussions on global health. Despite the various studies worldwide on pathophysiology, signs and symptoms, complications, and the best therapeutic option, the research is ongoing.

A persistence of symptoms for months has been observed in patients who had previously recovered from the disease. It was called prolonged COVID. The most frequent symptoms that persist are dyspnea, headache, dysgeusia, problems in the pattern of sleep, psychological problems—such as brain fog, anxiety, and depression. There are still vast unknowns, like how long residual post-COVID symptoms last and if they permanently affect the quality of life. Some authors comment that these symptoms decrease with time, a symptomatic treatment, and sometimes with the need for rehabilitation. In the reviewed literature, we did not find any other perspective to address the complications of COVID-19, in Mexico, besides the application of available treatments.

Since COVID is a disease that mainly affects the respiratory tract, its main complications are found in the lungs, taking into account the importance of comorbidities, which are considered the chief risk factor for the development of these, including patients with diabetes, hypertensive, or some cardiac pathology.

Conflict of interest

The authors declare no conflict of interest.

Author details

Efraín Navarro-Olivos[1], Gilberto Flores-Vargas[2], Guadalupe Irazú Morales-Reyes[2], Jéssica Paola Plascencia-Roldán[2], María de Jesús Gallardo-Luna[2] and Nicolás Padilla-Raygoza[2*]

1 Directorate of Teaching and Research, Institute of Public Health from Guanajuato State, Guanajuato, México

2 Department of Research and Technological Development, Directorate of Teaching and Research, Institute of Public Health from Guanajuato State, Guanajuato, México

*Address all correspondence to: npadillar@guanajuato.gob.mx

IntechOpen

© 2023 The Author(s). Licensee IntechOpen. This chapter is distributed under the terms of the Creative Commons Attribution License (http://creativecommons.org/licenses/by/3.0), which permits unrestricted use, distribution, and reproduction in any medium, provided the original work is properly cited.

References

[1] Zhu N, Zhang D, Wang W, Li X, Yang B, Song J, et al. A novel coronavirus from patients with pneumonia in China, 2019. The New England Journal of Medicine. 2020;**382**:727-733. DOI: 10.1056/NEJMoa2001017

[2] Hu B, Guo H, Zhou P, et al. Characteristics of SARS-CoV-2 and COVID-19. Nature Reviews. Microbiology. 2021;**19**:141-154. DOI: 10.1038/s41579-020-00459-7

[3] World Health Organization. Clinical management of severe acute respiratory infection (SARI) when COVID-19 disease is suspected. 2020. Available from: https://apps.who.int/iris/bitstream/handle/10665/331446/WHO-2019-nCoV-clinical-2020.4-eng.pdf?sequence=1&isAllowed=y

[4] Petrilli CM, Jones SA, Yang J, Rajagopalan H, O'Donnell L, Chernyak Y, et al. Factors associated with hospital admission and critical illness among 5279 people with coronavirus disease 2019 in new York City: Prospective cohort study. BMJ. 2020;**369**:m1966. DOI: 10.1136/bmj.m1966

[5] Xie J, Wu W, Liu S, Hu Y, Hu M, Li J, et al. Clinical characteristics and outcomes of critically ill patients with novel coronavirus infectious disease (COVID19) in China: A retrospective multicenter study. Intensive Care Medicine. 2020;**46**(10):1863-1872. DOI: 10.1007/s00134-020-06211-2

[6] Jiménez-Ruiz A, García-Grimshaw M, Ruiz-Sandoval JL. Manifestaciones neurológicas por COVID-19 Neurologic manifestations. Gaceta Médica de México. 2020;**156**(3). DOI: 10.24875/gmm.20000163

[7] Favas TT, Dev P, Chaurasia RN, Chakravarty K, Mishra R, Joshi D, et al. Neurological manifestations of COVID-19: A systematic review and meta-analysis of proportions. Neurological Sciences. 2020;**41**(12):3437-3470. DOI: 10.1007/s10072-020-04801-y

[8] Guadarrama-Ortiz P, Choreño-Parra JA, Sánchez-Martínez CM, Pacheco-Sánchez FJ, Rodríguez-Nava AI, García-Quintero G. Neurological aspects of SARS-CoV-2 infection: Mechanisms and manifestations. Frontiers in Neurology. 2020;**11**. DOI: 10.3389/fneur.2020.01039

[9] Zubair AS, McAlpine LS, Gardin T, Farhadian S, Kuruvilla DE, Spudich S. Neuropathogenesis and neurologic manifestations of the coronaviruses in the age of coronavirus disease 2019: A review. JAMA Neurology. 2020;**77**(8):1018-1027. DOI: 10.1001/jamaneurol.2020.2065

[10] Secretaria de Salud. Aviso Epidemiológico Enfermedad COVID-19 por SARS-CoV-2 (actualización). gob.mx. Available from: https://www.gob.mx/salud/documentos/aviso-epidemiologico-enfermedad-covid-19-por-sars-cov-2-actualizacion

[11] Carvalho T, Krammer F, Iwasaki A. The first 12 months of COVID-19: A timeline of immunological insights. Nature Reviews. Immunology. 2021;**21**(4):245-256. DOI: 10.1038/s41577-021-00522-1

[12] Secretaria de Salud. Informe Integral de COVID-19 en México. (Online). Mexico, Secretaria de Salud. 2022. Available from: https://coronavirus.gob.mx/wp-content/uploads/2022/02/Info-02-22-Int_COVID-19_26-enero-2022.pdf

[13] Wang H, Paulson KR, Pease SA, Watson S, Comfort H, Zheng P, et al.

Estimating excess mortality due to the COVID-19 pandemic: A systematic analysis of COVID-19-related mortality, 2020-21. The Lancet. 2022;**399**(10334):1513-1536

[14] Halabe-Cherem J, Robledo-Aburto Z, Fajardo-Dolci G. Síndrome Post-Covid, Certezas e Interrogantes. 1th. ed. Ciudad de México: Panamericana; 2022. Available from: https://anmm.org.mx/publicaciones/ultimas_publicaciones/Libro-Sindrome-post-COVID.pdf

[15] Michelen M, Manoharan L, Elkheir N, Cheng V, Dagens A, Hastie C, et al. Characterising long COVID: A living systematic review. BMJ Global Health. 2021;**6**(9):e005427. DOI: 10.1136/bmjgh-2021-005427

[16] Choutka J, Jansari V, Hornig M, Iwasaki A. Unexplained post-acute infection syndromes. Nature Medicine. 2022;**28**(5):911-923. DOI: 10.1038/s41591-022-01810-6

[17] Gaebler C, Wang Z, Lorenzi JCC, Muecksch F, Finkin S, Tokuyama M, et al. Evolution of antibody immunity to SARS-CoV-2. Nature. 2021;**591**(7851):639-644. DOI: 10.1038/s41586-021-03207-w

[18] Wallukat G, Hohberger B, Wenzel K, Fürst J, Schulze-Rothe S, Wallukat A, et al. Functional autoantibodies against G-protein coupled receptors in patients with persistent long-COVID-19 symptoms. Journal of Translational Autoimmunity. 2021;**4**:100100. DOI: 10.1016/j.jtauto.2021.100100

[19] Office for Civil Rights (OCR). Guidance on "long COVID" as a disability under the ADA, section 504, and section 1557. HHS.gov. US Department of Health and Human Services; 2021. Available from: https://www.hhs.gov/civil-rights/for-providers/civil-rights-covid19/guidance-long-covid-disability/index.html

[20] Torres-Cuevas L, Gil-Guzmán OA, Torres-Escalante JL, Luis J. Potenciales secuelas en la salud por Covid-19 en México: ¿Qué debemos de esperar? Archivos en Medicina Familiar. 2022;**24**(1):67-73. Available from: https://www.medigraphic.com/pdfs/medfam/amf-2022/amf221i.pdf

[21] Blagojevic NR, Bosnjakovic D, Vukomanovic V, Arsenovic S, Lazic JS, Tadic M. Acute pericarditis and severe acute respiratory syndrome coronavirus 2: Case report. International Journal of Infectious Diseases. 2020;**101**:180-182. DOI: 10.1016/j.ijid.2020.09.1440

[22] Osman W, Ahmed A, Elawad O, Albashir A. A case of acute pericarditis and subsequent pericardial effusion in COVID-19 patient: A case report. Authorea. 2020. DOI: 10.22541/au.159969834.49964606

[23] Wong Chew RM, Ángel Ambrocio AH, Bautista Carbajal P, García León ML, Vite Velázquez X, Cortázar Maldonado LA, et al. Efectos a largo plazo de la COVID-19: una revisión de la literatura. Acta Médica Grupo Ángeles. 2021;**19**(3):421-428. DOI: 10.35366/101741

[24] Flores-Silva FD, García-Grimshaw M, Valdés-Ferrer SI, Vigueras-Hernández AP, Domínguez-Moreno R, Tristán-Samaniego DP, et al. Neurologic manifestations in hospitalized patients with COVID-19 in Mexico City. PLoS One. 2021;**16**(4). DOI: 10.1371/journal.pone.0247433

[25] Albarran-Sanchez A, Noyola-García ME, Calderón-Vallejo A, Guízar-García LA, Rosales-Dueñas FJ, Barrientos-Flores CJ, et al. Manifestaciones neurológicas en pacientes con COVID-19 severo en un centro de tercer

nivel de atención. Revista Médica del Instituto Mexicano del Seguro Social. 2021;**596**:545-550. Available from: https://pubmed.ncbi.nlm.nih.gov/34910416/

[26] Villalpando JMG, Forcelledo HA, Castillo JLB, Sastré AJ, Rojop IEJ, Hernández VO, et al. COVID-19, long COVID syndrome, and mental health sequelae in a Mexican population. International Journal of Environmental Research and Public Health. 2022;**19**(12):6970. DOI: 10.3390/ijerph19126970

[27] Jing Y, Run-Qian L, Hao-Ran W, Hao-Ran C, Ya-Bin L, Yang G, et al. Potential influence of COVID-19/ACE2 on the female reproductive system. Molecular Human Reproduction. 2020;**26**(6):367-373. DOI: 10.1093/molehr/gaaa030

[28] Batiha O, Al-Deeb T, Al-Zoubi E, Alsharu E. Impact of COVID-19 and other viruses on reproductive health. Andrologia. 2020;**52**(9):e13791. DOI: 10.1111/and.13791

[29] Verma S, Saksena S, Sadri-Ardekani H. ACE2 receptor expression in testes: Implications in coronavirus disease 2019 pathogenesis. Biology of Reproduction. 2020;**103**(3):449-451. DOI: 10.1093/biolre/ioaa080

[30] Davis HE, Assaf GS, McCorkell L, Wei H, Low RJ, Re'em Y, et al. Characterizing long COVID in an international cohort: 7 months of symptoms and their impact. EClinicalMedicine. 2021;**38**:101019. DOI: 10.1016/j.eclinm.2021.101019

[31] Guía Clínica para la Atención del Paciente Long Covid/Covid Persistente. 2021. Inmunologia.org. Available from: https://www.inmunologia.org/images/site/GUIA_consenso_COVID_persistente.pdf

[32] Borromeo S, Gomez-Calero C, Molina E, Fernández-Huerte J, Martínez-Monge N, Muñoz AT, et al. Objective Assessment of a New Olfactory Rehabilitation Approach in Adults with Olfactory Impairments Using Functional Magnetic Resonance (fMRI). Converging Clinical and Engineering Research on Neurorehabiliatation. Berlín, Heidelberg: Springer Berlin Heidelberg; 2013. pp. 381-384. DOI: 10.1007/978-3-642-34546-3_61

[33] Alvarez-Moreno CA, Pineda J, Bareño A, Espitia R, Rengifo P. Long COVID-19 in Latin America: Low prevalence, high resilience or low surveillance and difficulties accessing health care? Travel Medicine and Infectious Disease. 2023;**51**:102492. DOI: 10.1016/j.tmaid.2022.102492

[34] González-Hermosillo JA, Martínez-López JP, Carrillo-Lampón SA, Ruiz-Ojeda D, Herrera-Ramírez S, Amezcua-Guerra LM, et al. Post-acute COVID-19 symptoms, a potential link with Myalgic encephalomyelitis/chronic fatigue syndrome: A 6-month survey in a Mexican cohort. Brain Sciences. 2021;**11**(6):760. DOI: 10.3390/brainsci11060760